Working with Voice Disorders

T0144083

Now in a fully revised and updated third edition, *Working with Voice Disorders* offers practical insight and direction into all aspects of voice disorders, from assessment and diagnosis to intervention and case management. Using evidence-based material, it provides clinicians with pragmatic, accessible support, facilitating and informing decision-making along the clinical journey, from referral to discharge.

Key features of this resource include:

- A wealth of new, up-to-date practical and theoretical information, covering topics such as the prevention, assessment, intervention and treatment of a wide spectrum of voice disorders.
- A multi-dimensional structure, allowing the clinician to consider both specific aspects of patient management and aspects such as clinical effectiveness, clinical efficiencies and service management.
- Photocopiable clinical resources, from an at-a-glance summary of voice disorders to treatment and assessment protocols, and practical exercises and advice sheets for patients.
- Sample programmes for voice information groups and teacher workshops.
- Checklists for patients on topics such as the environmental and acoustic challenges of the workplace.
- Self-assessed personalised voice review sheets and weekly voice diaries encourage patients to monitor their voice quality and utilise strategies to prevent vocal misuse.

Combining the successful format of mixing theory and practice, this edition offers a patient-centred approach to voice disorders in a fully accessible and easy-to-read format and addresses the challenges of service provision in a changing world. This is an essential resource for speech and language therapists of varying levels of experience, from student to specialist.

Stephanie Martin's career as a speech and language therapist combined clinical practice, research, lecturing, student supervision and writing. She holds an MA in Voice Studies and was awarded a doctorate for her research exploring factors which have an impact on the vocal performance and vocal effectiveness of newly qualified teachers and lecturers.

Stephanie is a Past-President of the British Voice Association and in 2005 was awarded Fellowship of the Royal College of Speech and Language Therapists (RCSLT) for research and teaching. She represented the RCSLT for three years as a member of the Standing Liaison Committee of Speech and Language Therapists Logopedists in the European Union.

In addition to the strong clinical bias of her publications with Myra Lockhart, *The Voice Sourcebook* began a writing partnership with Lyn Darnley drawn from their workshops, addressing issues with the teacher's voice. Their most recent publication, *The Voice in Education*, was published in 2019.

The *Working With* Series

The *Working With* series provides speech and language therapists with a range of 'go-to' resources, full of well-sourced, up-to-date information regarding specific disorders. Underpinned by robust theoretical foundations and supported by intervention options and exercises, every book ensures that the reader has access to the latest thinking regarding diagnosis, management and treatment options.

Written in a fully accessible style, each book bridges theory and practice and offers ready-to-use and well-rehearsed practical material, including guidance on interventions, management advice, and therapeutic resources for the client, parent or carer. The series is an invaluable resource for practitioners, whether speech and language therapy students, or more experienced clinicians.

Books in the series include:

Working with Voice Disorders
Theory and Practice, Third Edition
Stephanie Martin
2021/pb: 9780367331634

Working with Voice Disorders

Theory and Practice

Third Edition

Stephanie Martin

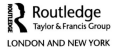
Routledge
Taylor & Francis Group

LONDON AND NEW YORK

Third edition published 2021
by Routledge
2 Park Square, Milton Park, Abingdon, Oxon OX14 4RN

and by Routledge
52 Vanderbilt Avenue, New York, NY 10017

Routledge is an imprint of the Taylor & Francis Group, an informa business

© 2021 Stephanie Martin

The right of Stephanie Martin to be identified as author of this work has been asserted by her in accordance with sections 77 and 78 of the Copyright, Designs and Patents Act 1988.

All rights reserved. The purchase of this copyright material confers the right on the purchasing institution to photocopy or download pages which bear the companion website icon and a copyright line at the bottom of the page. No other parts of this book may be reprinted or reproduced or utilised in any form or by any electronic, mechanical, or other means, now known or hereafter invented, including photocopying and recording, or in any information storage or retrieval system, without permission in writing from the publishers.

Trademark notice: Product or corporate names may be trademarks or registered trademarks, and are used only for identification and explanation without intent to infringe.

First edition published by Speechmark Publishing Ltd 2000
Second edition published by Speechmark Publishing Ltd 2013

British Library Cataloguing-in-Publication Data
A catalogue record for this book is available from the British Library

Library of Congress Cataloging-in-Publication Data
Names: Martin, Stephanie, author. Title: Working with voice disorders : theory and practice / Stephanie Martin. Description: Third edition. | Abingdon, Oxon; New York, NY: Routledge, [2021] | Series: Working with | Includes bibliographical references and index.
Identifiers: LCCN 2020029767 (print) | LCCN 2020029768 (ebook) |
ISBN 9780367636272 (hardback) | ISBN 9780367331634 (paperback) |
ISBN 9780429318221 (ebook)
Subjects: LCSH: Voice disorders–Treatment. | Speech therapy.
Classification: LCC RF510.M37 2021 (print) | LCC RF510 (ebook) | DDC 616.85/56–dc23
LC record available at https://lccn.loc.gov/2020029767
LC ebook record available at https://lccn.loc.gov/2020029768

ISBN: 978-0-367-63627-2 (hbk)
ISBN: 978-0-367-33163-4 (pbk)
ISBN: 978-0-429-31822-1 (ebk)

Typeset in Interstate
by Newgen Publishing UK

Visit the companion website: www.routledge.com/cw/speechmark

Contents

Acknowledgements

I very much wish to acknowledge the support, encouragement and generosity received over many years from friends, colleagues, students and patients who added and continue to add to my understanding of, and experience in, the field of voice.

The influence of two people in the writing of this book must have particular mention. Long-term colleague and friend, Myra Lockhart, contributed her knowledge, wisdom and clinical expertise as co-author of the two previous editions of *Working with Voice Disorders*. This edition has been extensively rewritten without her input, but has built on the firm foundation developed through our previous writing partnership; on this occasion I have missed her wise counsel and valuable input.

Lyn Darnley, whose work and doctoral research focused on theatre voice and actor training, has been a colleague and friend of many years' standing, and her skill in and knowledge of practical voice is without equal and generously shared. My knowledge and practical voice skills have developed immeasurably over many years of working with Lyn in the field of the teachers' voice, which has been both absorbing and fulfilling.

To them all and particularly to my family, I give my heartfelt thanks.

To my immense sadness, Lyn died shortly after the completion of this publication. Through her teaching and writing she leaves a lasting legacy to the worldwide voice community.

Figures

Tables

INTRODUCTION

Working with Voice Disorders has been written for students in training and practicing clinicians, indeed for all those professionals who have an interest in and work together for the benefit of the patient with voice disorders. This book is essentially a practical resource, grounded in theory and addressing all aspects of patient management from assessment to service delivery. Voice is a critical indicator of both physiological and psychological well-being and as such offers a particularly effective gauge of physical and mental health. This relationship between the patient and their voice is an essential component in both differential diagnosis and intervention.

The book explores the course of the patient's journey, preparing the clinician for the issues intrinsic to voice disorders. It includes an overview of the anatomy and physiology of voice and describes the spectrum of voice disorders. It leads the clinician through assessment, case-history taking, treatment planning, intervention, practical management strategies and service delivery. While its presentation mirrors the course of the care episode, readers may simply wish to refer to specific areas of personal interest. Although intended to be read in its entirety, each chapter deals with discrete topics, which allow the reader to self-select.

The structure and philosophy of this extensively revised edition of *Working with Voice Disorders* retains much of the organisation of the previous editions. It contains a wealth of updated practical and theoretical information, from the at-a-glance summary of voice disorders to a complete treatment programme, including exercises, sample proforma, patient checklists and advice sheets plus workshop outlines, all of which can be freely copied for clinical use. As with all dynamic areas of medicine, change is continuous and the world of voice is not immune to change. Changes to instrumentation, surgical intervention, new discoveries in histology, increased collaborative working, the challenges of the COVID-19 pandemic, the future shape of the world of voice in terms of service provision are all addressed. One ingredient is missing, that of Myra Lockhart, who co-authored the previous editions; all errors and omissions are my own.

It is hoped that the book will fulfil its intended purpose, that of providing an invaluable resource for every clinician, increasing their confidence and competence in a field which has absorbed the author for many years.

ANATOMY OVERVIEW

Introduction

This chapter is intended principally as a brief overview of the anatomy, physiology and neuroanatomy of 'voice production'. For those readers who are looking for very detailed information there are many widely available excellent resources, both publications and online. The purpose of this chapter is, however, to offer an easily accessible overview for readers outlining the structures and functions central to the production of voice and noting how they change over time.

The process of producing voice

Voice production is dependent on three different, but interrelated, systems:

- the respiratory system – responsible for the manner and pattern of breathing;
- the phonatory system – responsible for how sound is produced at the level of the larynx;
- the resonatory system – responsible for the modification of the sound.

These separate but interconnecting systems have been adapted to work together in the process of voice production, although their primary biological purpose is, of course, to assist in life support.

While recognition is given to the interdependence of the three systems, for the purpose of this chapter each system will be differentiated, one from the other. It is, however, important to remember that vocal quality changes are part of a composite and nuanced picture. Vocal quality changes that are recognised as disordered or different are often the result of cumulative changes within each system. Each system has its own individual and separate identity, but a change in one system may precipitate change in another, so a principal 'cause' of the disorder may be difficult to establish. Mathieson (2001) suggests that when a physiological change occurs in the larynx, a pathological change may well have been the precipitating feature, or indeed pathological change may be the result of physiological change, a view with which the author strongly concurs.

The respiratory system

The main purpose of the respiratory system is to maintain life by carrying air into the lungs where the exchange of gases, oxygen and carbon dioxide takes place.

Oxygen enters the bloodstream and excess carbon dioxide moves out through the capillaries surrounding the alveoli within the lungs. The respiratory system can be said to begin at the nose and the mouth, and end with the alveoli in the lungs. Within this system two distinctive respiratory tracts are identified. The upper respiratory tract is composed of the nasal and oral cavities, the pharynx and the larynx. In addition to its role in respiration, the upper respiratory tract has multiple functions, such as the processes of chewing, swallowing, articulation, resonance and phonation. The lower respiratory tract refers to the trachea, the bronchi and lungs, which are housed within the bony thoracic skeleton or ribcage, and in contrast to the upper respiratory tract, functions exclusively for the process of breathing for life and for phonation.

The upper and lower respiratory tracts comprise the vocal tract and, as may be surmised by their close alignment, are functionally interdependent so that modifications to one will affect the function of the other.

The respiratory tract has two parallel entrances, the nose and the mouth, through which air enters. These entrances merge into a common tract, known as the pharynx. The pharynx is a cone-shaped tube approximately 13–14 cm long, composed of muscular and membranous layers, wider at the top where it is continuous with the nasal cavity and opening laterally into the mouth. At its lower and narrower end it leads into the laryngeal inlet anteriorly and the oesophagus posteriorly. The area within the pharynx immediately behind the nose (the nasopharynx) and the area behind the mouth (the oropharynx) are separated by a muscular valve, the soft palate, which, when raised, closes off one section from the other, thus effectively preventing food or liquid escaping from the nose when swallowing. Along with the most inferior part of the pharynx, which contracts at rest and prevents any reflux of the stomach contents into the pharynx or air entering the oesophagus, the soft palate forms part of the involuntary protective mechanism in the respiratory tract. By far the most vigorous protective mechanisms, which are involuntary and reflexive, exist within the larynx. Some mechanisms attempt to 'repel' by closing off the airway and some attempt to 'expel' by forcing substances out of the respiratory tract.

The respiratory tract, passing through the laryngeal inlet, continues into the trachea, which divides into two branches, and subsequently into the smaller bronchi that enter the lungs, and ultimately into the alveoli. Protective mechanisms exist along the respiratory tract to prevent inadvertent damage; for example, the lungs are encased by the bony thoracic skeleton, or ribcage, consisting of 12 pairs of ribs. Each set of ribs has different dimensions and degrees of flexibility of movement.

The first pair is the shortest (the paired ribs increase in length up to rib 7 and then decrease in length up to rib 12) and immobile, fused to the breastbone or sternum at the front and at the back to the spinal vertebrae. Pairs two to seven are similarly attached, but by synovial joints which permit a degree of rotation, while pairs eight to ten are attached to each other at the front by flexible cartilage. Pairs 11 and 12 (sometimes referred to as 'floating ribs') are fixed at the back to the spinal vertebrae but have no fixed attachment at the front to the sternum. The somewhat idiosyncratic arrangement of the ribs is important, in that the pleural or membranous connection between the lungs and thoracic cavity allows expansion and contraction of this area as a single unit and along three planes for inspiration and expiration. During inspiration the vertical dimension is increased by contraction of the diaphragm, the upward movement of the ribs increases the transverse diameter while a simultaneous forward and upward movement of the sternum increases the antero-posterior diameter. The orientation of the ribs controls their mobility and this flexible cavity, which also contains major organs such as the heart, the aorta and vena cava, the trachea and oesophagus, can then accommodate changes in the size of the pear-shaped lungs, which expand to contain greater amounts of air when needed to support speech or song. Modification of the respiratory cycle to quick intake and slow release of air, which is essential for this process, may be contrasted with the equal phases of inspiration and expiration common to quiet, at rest, breathing for life, which is predominately under medullary control and heavily influenced by the level of carbon dioxide present in a particular environment (Table 1.1).

The muscles of respiration have clearly defined roles and most are concerned either with inspiration (Figure 1.1) or expiration (Figure 1.2), but some, like the latissimus dorsi (the largest muscle in the upper body) have a more overarching function within respiration and are concerned with both inspiration and expiration.

In resting respiration, air is inspired at approximately a dozen times per minute, but this muscular activity goes largely unnoticed despite the fact that there is active muscular contraction to enlarge the thorax. The diaphragm and the external intercostals are most responsible for this activity. For the purposes of speech and song, inspiration needs to be more vigorous and, to this end, accessory muscles are recruited to help the diaphragm and external intercostals increase thoracic volume. The volume of air inspired and the effort exerted will, of course, vary depending on the demands made.

For the purposes of this brief overview the following provides an at-a-glance guide to the muscles involved in inspiration and expiration.

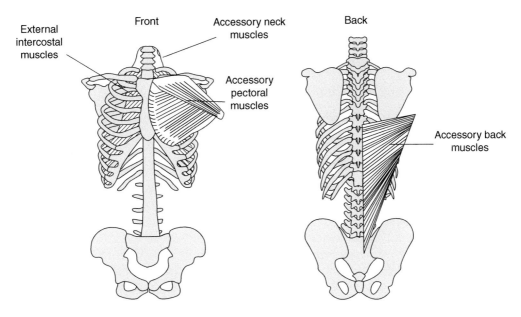

Front

External intercostal muscles

Accessory neck muscles

Accessory pectoral muscles

Back

Accessory back muscles

Figure 1.1 Muscles of inspiration

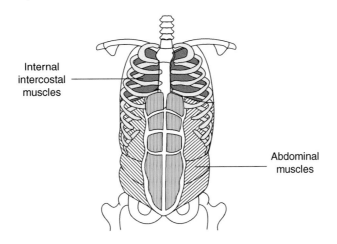

Internal intercostal muscles

Abdominal muscles

Figure 1.2 Muscles of expiration

Principal muscles of inspiration

The diaphragm – this large, dome-shaped involuntary muscle is of great importance in respiration. During sleep and unconsciousness it maintains respiration under involuntary control.

The external intercostal muscles – these muscles act to control the amount of space between the ribs and aid air intake.

Accessory muscles of inspiration

The sternocleidomastoid and scalene muscle group – these are accessory neck muscles which help to elevate the first and second ribs during inspiration.

The serratus posterior superior, latissimus dorsi and levatores costarum – these are accessory back muscles which contribute to rib movement during inspiration.

The pectoralis major and minor, the serratus anterior and the subclavious muscles – these are accessory pectoral muscles which contribute to the expansion of the upper ribcage.

The accessory muscles of inspiration are not usually recruited during normal respiration but may be accessed during prolonged exercise or in individuals with, for example, chronic obstructive pulmonary disease (COPD) or severe asthma.

Muscles of expiration

As with inspiration there are two types of expiration – passive and active. With passive expiration, expiration above the resting expiratory level usually is accomplished not by muscular effort but by non-muscular forces that may be said to be the result of the elastic recoil of the lungs. For controlled active expiration, in particular for increasing intensity or duration of sound, muscular activity is necessary over and above elastic recoil to reduce the volumes of the lungs and thorax. Two different muscle processes are involved to support active expiration: muscles that contract alternatively to the diaphragm and support expiration, and muscles that lower the ribcage.

Muscles that aid active expiration

The rectus abdominis, external and internal oblique and the transversus abdominis are the abdominal muscles responsible for a decrease in the dimensions of the thoracic cavity. Their action increases intra-abdominal pressure, causing the abdominal contents to push upward and inward against the diaphragm, forcing it to return to its relaxed position and helping air to flow out of the lungs. The internal intercostal muscles contract to pull the ribs downwards and stiffen the rib interspaces. The transversus thoracic, the sub-costals, the quadratus lumborum and the serratus posterior inferior are accessory back muscles which exert a downward pull on the ribs.

As a brief summary, the muscular effort involved in the cycle of respiration is shown in Table 1.1.

Innervation of the respiratory system

As has already been stated, the muscles of the respiratory system are under both voluntary and involuntary control. Vegetative breathing, or resting breathing, already discussed, is primarily under involuntary control while breathing for speech or non-speech activities is the result of voluntary and involuntary influences.

Table 1.1 Cycle of respiration

Phase	Muscles involved
Inspiration	Abdominal muscles and internal intercostals relax. External intercostals contract to fully expand the rib cage. Diaphragm contracts and descends which enlarges the lung space
Expiration – Stage 1	Without muscular effort to keep rib cage expanded it 'relaxes' back to rest position, known as 'elastic recoil', which initiates airflow
Expiration – Stage 2	Contraction of the internal intercostals added to last of 'elastic recoil' adds to lung pressure
Expiration – Stage 3	Abdominal muscles used to provide the final possible amount of lung pressure

Table 1.2 Muscles of inspiration

Muscles of inspiration	Innervation
Diaphragm	Phrenic nerve C3–C5
External intercostals	Intercostal nerves
Sternocleidomastoid	Spinal accessory
Scaleni	C4–C6
Latissimus dorsi	C6, C7 and C8
Pectoralis major	Medial and lateral anterior thoracic nerves
Pectoralis minor	Brachial plexus

Table 1.3 Muscles of expiration

Muscles of expiration	Innervation
Rectus abdominis	T6 to T12
External and internal oblique	T6 to T12
Transversus abdominis	T7 to T12
Internal intercostals	T2 to T12

The nerves that innervate voluntary movement of the muscles of respiration are shown in Tables 1.2 and 1.3.

Role of respiration

The role of respiration in speech is of paramount importance, as within the broad spectrum of physiological function in speech, respiration is involved in the regulation of parameters such as intensity, fundamental frequency, linguistic stress and the division of speech into various units. Information on lung volume and lung capacity measurement is summarised below, but it should be remembered that lung capacity varies considerably among individuals and is affected by a number of factors, among which are age, gender, size, weight, physical condition and health. Many clinicians do not feel that the inclusion of lung volume and lung capacity measures are necessary as part of respiratory function profiling, providing the patient is able to maintain adequate air volume and airflow for speech; of more value is information relating to the control of the respiratory system during speech. A caveat to that is that analysis of respiratory function is considered very helpful for professional voice users, singers and actors. The tidal volume of air used for respiration or voice is rarely fully used, often only 10–15% of the tidal volume is used, but for demanding physical activities and singing the entire tidal volume may be required. For that reason, clinicians may want to be selective in so far as the assessment of respiratory function is concerned with reference to specific client groups.

Lung volumes

The four lung volumes are as follows:

- Tidal Volume (TV) is the amount of air inspired or expired during a respiratory cycle at rest.
- Inspiratory Reserve Volume (IRV) is the maximum amount of air that can be taken into the lungs beyond the end of tidal inspiration.
- Expiratory Reserve Volume (ERV) is the greatest volume of air that can be expired at the end of spontaneous expiration.
- Residual Volume (RV) is the amount of air that remains in the lungs and airways at the end of maximal expiration.

Lung capacities

The four lung capacities are as follows:

- Vital Capacity (VC) is the greatest amount of air that can be expelled from the lungs and airways after maximal inspiration.
- The maximum Tidal Volume (TV) of air that can be held in the lungs excluding residual is on average 4.25–6.25 litres in the male and 2.1–4.25 litres in the female.
- Functional Residual Capacity (FRC) is the volume of air contained within the lungs and airways at the resting expiratory level.
- Total Lung Capacity (TLC) is the volume of air contained within the lungs and airways at the end of maximal inspiration.

The phonatory system

The phonatory system consists of the larynx, its extrinsic and intrinsic muscles and cartilages and the hyoid bone which, although not actually part of the larynx, has an important role as many of the extrinsic muscles of the larynx have an attachment to it. It goes without saying that treatment of the voice-disordered patient demands knowledge far beyond that of laryngeal anatomy and the recognition of various pathologies, but it is essential that the interdependence of anatomy, physiology, neurology and acoustics should form the cornerstone of clinical thinking. The concern of this chapter, however, is to offer a brief overview of the anatomy of the larynx, an explanation of its structure and how it functions in voice production.

The principal biological function of the larynx is to act as a protective life-saving mechanism within the respiratory tract, acting as a valve which both prevents foreign substances from entering the larynx and expels those that bypass the system. The effective laryngeal valving mechanism, which is achieved through the coordinated action of the intrinsic and extrinsic laryngeal muscles, elevates intra-thoracic pressure, which aids weight-bearing, lifting, coughing, defecation and childbirth. It is worth saying that these strong vegetative functions of the larynx should be considered during the diagnostic process as they may often contribute to a voice disorder through, for example, damage or trauma to the vocal fold mucosa as a result of excessive coughing or the extreme tension that the vocal folds endure when firmly adducted during any form of strenuous weight-bearing exertion, such as working out in a gym to develop upper body strength or training with fixed weights.

Structure of the larynx

Cartilages of the larynx

The larynx is made up of nine individual cartilages: three large single cartilages – the thyroid, cricoid and epiglottis, and three smaller paired cartilages – the arytenoid, corniculate and cuneiform cartilages (Figure 1.3). For the purposes of voice the most important are the thyroid, cricoid, epiglottis and arytenoid. Cartilage, which is softer and more flexible than

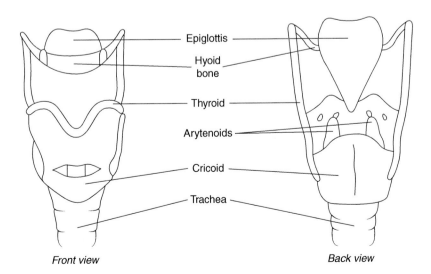

Front view   Back view

Figure 1.3 Cartilages of the larynx

bone, is made from chondrocyte cells and an intercellular substance containing mucopoly-saccharide sulphate and fibres. Hyaline cartilage differs from elastic cartilage in that the fibres are thin, dense and collagenous, whereas elastic cartilage fibres are dense and, as their name suggests, elastic.

The thyroid cartilage

The thyroid cartilage is the largest cartilage, which forms most of the anterior and lateral walls of the larynx. Shaped like a shield, it is essentially composed of two quadrilateral plates of hyaline cartilage, the thyroid laminae, which are fused at the midline anteriorly at a peak known as the laryngeal prominence or Adam's apple. The degree at which the plates meet varies between men and women, approximately 120 degrees in women and children but 90 degrees post puberty in men, which explains the very pronounced outline of this cartilage in the male. The thyroid laminae protect the vocal folds, which extend across the laryngeal space from the inside of the thyroid cartilage to the arytenoid cartilages. The posterior border of each plate is prolonged upwards and downwards as cornu – the superior and inferior horns, respectively. Muscular attachments (see below) link the superior horn with the hyoid bone and the inferior horn with the cricoid cartilage.

The cricoid cartilage

The second largest cartilage, the cricoid cartilage, is also composed of hyaline cartilage. Located immediately above the trachea, it is narrow anteriorly and broad and flat poster-iorly, articulates with the thyroid cartilage on its posterolateral surface and forms the base of the larynx. It is the only circumferential structure in the larynx. On its lateral margins there are two articulate facets into which fit the inferior horns of the thyroid.

The epiglottis

The epiglottis is a broad, leaf-shaped elastic cartilage, attached to the medial surface of the thyroid cartilage. The anterior surface is attached via a ligament to the hyoid bone. The epiglottis does not function in the production of voice – its main purpose is as another protective mechanism to prevent food from entering the larynx. It may, however, modify laryngeal tone by alterations in the size and shape of the pharyngeal cavity. This is as a consequence of positional changes it makes as a result of tongue movements.

The arytenoid cartilages

The arytenoid cartilages are small, paired, pyramidal-shaped cartilages with three pronounced angles, made of hyaline and elastic cartilaginous material, that articulate with the cricoid cartilage via the cricoarytenoid joints. The specialised nature of this synovial joint allows rocking and gliding movements of the arytenoids. These vocal gymnasts they can glide medially

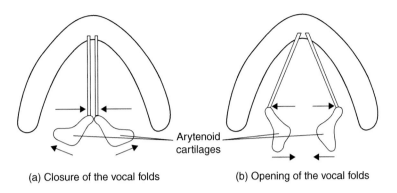

(a) Closure of the vocal folds   (b) Opening of the vocal folds

Figure 1.4 Schematic illustration of the movement of the arytenoids cartilages and consequent movement of the vocal folds

and laterally, rotate slightly, and may also slide forwards and backwards, but with restricted movement. Almost any combination of the above movements may occur simultaneously. The base of the arytenoid has two extensions: the anterior one, the vocal process, which forms the point of insertion for the vocal folds (allowing the vocal folds to open and close with ease and thus produce changes in pitch), and the posterolateral extension, or muscular process to which the posterior cricoarytenoid and lateral arytenoid muscles attach (Figure 1.4).

The corniculate and cuneiform cartilages

The corniculate are two small conical elastic cartilages at the apex of the arytenoid cartilages. The tiny, club- or rod-shaped cuneiform cartilages, when present, are contained within the aryepiglottic folds (a fold of tissue which extends from the arytenoids to the epi-glottis). There is frequent normal variation in these cartilages which do not appear to have any clinical significance and currently neither the corniculate nor the cuneiform cartilages appear to have a reported role in laryngeal function.

The hyoid bone

Shaped like a horseshoe, the hyoid bone is situated in the anterior midline of the neck superior to the thyroid cartilage. As previously mentioned, although the hyoid bone is not strictly part of the larynx, it is anchored by muscles from anterior, posterior and inferior directions. The hyoid provides attachment to the muscles of the floor of the mouth and the tongue above, the larynx below and the epiglottis and pharynx behind and indeed to the skull base by muscles and ligaments (see extrinsic muscles of the larynx below).

Muscles of the larynx

The muscles of the larynx may be divided into extrinsic and intrinsic muscle groups. The extrinsic muscles have one point of attachment to a structure within the larynx and one point of attachment to a structure outside the larynx. Their function is to position the larynx within the vocal tract, either fixing, raising or lowering it. The intrinsic muscles have both points of attachment to structures within the larynx. They are concerned with fine movement of the vocal folds for phonation, for respiration, for containing air below the glottis and for assisting in the protective mechanism of preventing food or liquid being ingested during swallowing.

Extrinsic muscles of the larynx

The larynx is innervated by branches of the vague nerve on each side. Sensory innervations to the glottis and laryngeal vestibule is by the internal branch of the superior laryngeal nerve. The external branch of the superior laryngeal nerve innervates the cricothyroid muscles. There are eight extrinsic muscles, four of which lie above the level of the hyoid – the suprahyoid muscles, which act principally to elevate the larynx and support the hyoid bone. Four lie below the hyoid – the infrahyoid muscles, which act as laryngeal depressors. The latter are particularly important in lengthening the vocal tract, which has a significant effect on vocal resonance. Detailed descriptions of the extrinsic laryngeal muscles can be found in a number of texts, but for the purposes of this chapter an outline of the muscles, their function and innervation are given in Table 1.4.

Voice production is dependent upon a fine balance between the force exerted by air pressure as it is exhaled from the lungs and the resistance of the intrinsic muscles of the larynx. Intrinsic laryngeal muscles (ILM) are highly specialised muscles involved in phonation and airway protection, with unique properties that allow them to perform extremely rapid contractions for a prolonged period (Figure 1.5). It has been hypothesised that they may differ from limb muscles in several physiological aspects and it has been suggested

Table 1.4 Extrinsic muscles of the larynx

	Function	Innervation
Suprahyoid muscles		
Digastric	Raises the hyoid bone Depresses mandible	Anterior CN5; Posterior CN7
Mylohyoid	Raises floor of mouth Depresses mandible Pulls hyoid forward	CN5
Stylohyoid	Raises hyoid Pulls hyoid backwards	CN 7
Geniohyoid	Raises hyoid Pulls it forward Depresses mandible	CN 1
Infrahyoid muscles		
Thyrohyoid	Pulls hyoid bone and thyroid cartilages together	Hypoglossal CN1
Sternothyroid	Draws the larynx down	Ansa cervicalis C1-C3
Sternohyoid	Depresses hyoid bone	Ansa cervicalis C1-C3
Omohyoid	Depresses hyoid bone	Ansa cervicalis C1-C3

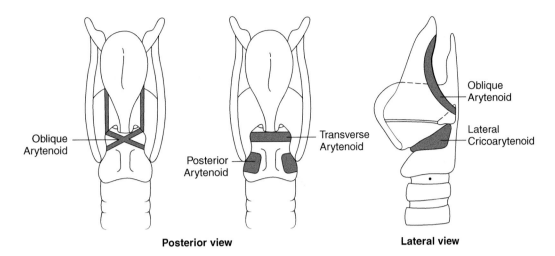

Figure 1.5 Cross-section of larynx showing intrinsic muscles

(Ferretti *et al.*, 2015) that the profile of the proteins that regulate calcium levels in ILM explains their unique properties.

The chief muscles within this group (see below), named after the cartilages to which they are attached, are all capable of independent movement but often work synergistically during vocalisation. Increased or imbalanced tension of the intrinsic and/or the extrinsic laryngeal muscles may modify the configuration of the vocal tract (Yamasaki *et al.*, 2011). In their study of adult female patients with vocal nodules the authors noted significant differences in the vocal tract morphometry of individuals with vocal nodules when compared with normal female adult subjects at rest. For example, a reduction in the laryngeal vestibule area which was significantly smaller in the dysphonic group, the distance between the right and left vocal processes of the arytenoid cartilages, and the distance between the anterior commissure of the glottis and the laryngeal posterior wall were also significantly lower in the dysphonic group.

The thyroarytenoid muscles

The thyroarytenoid muscles are paired muscles that extend from the inner surface of the thyroid cartilage to the arytenoid cartilages and comprise the bulk of the vocal folds. On contraction they decrease the length and longitudinal tension of the vocal fold and increase vocal fold mass. They are important in the production of low vocal pitch, and as they actively change the configuration of the vocal folds themselves there will be a resultant change in the way in which they move within the vibratory cycle.

The cricothyroid muscles

The cricothyroid muscles are considered to be the only tensor muscles of the larynx and the main muscles for controlling pitch as they extend from the upper surface of the cricoid cartilage to the lower border of the thyroid cartilage. On contraction, they tilt the thyroid forward, thus increasing the distance between the thyroid cartilage and the vocal process of the arytenoids. As a result, the vocal folds are stretched, which thins the vocal folds and sharpens their edges, allowing them to vibrate at higher frequencies and leading to a perception of increased pitch.

The posterior cricoarytenoids

The posterior cricoarytenoids are paired muscles extending from the posterior lamina of the cricoid to the muscular process of the arytenoids. Their action is one of rotation and separation of the arytenoids and as a result they abduct the vocal folds. It has long been considered that they are the only intrinsic muscles in the larynx that do so, although that is a view that has, however, been challenged by those who consider that the lateral cricoarytenoid muscles could also have a role in abduction of the vocal folds.

The interarytenoid muscles

The interarytenoid muscles is the collective name given to the transverse arytenoid and the oblique arytenoid. The transverse arytenoid connects one arytenoid to the other while the oblique arytenoid extends from the muscular process of one arytenoid to the apex of the other and then upwards into the lateral margin of the epiglottis. These muscles adduct the vocal folds (Table 1.5).

The lateral cricoarytenoids

The lateral cricoarytenoids are paired muscles arising from the sides and upper surface of the cricoid cartilage to the muscle process of the arytenoids. Functioning together with the interarytenoids they adduct the vocal folds. The close interrelationship of the posterior cricoarytenoid muscles and the lateral cricoarytenoids might, as already noted, suggest that they too have a role in the abduction of the vocal folds.

Table 1.5 Intrinsic muscles of the larynx

Muscle	Function	Innervation
Cricothyroid	Increases length and tension of vocal folds	Vagus (superior laryngeal branch)
Thyroarytenoid	Increases tension and mass of the vocal folds	Vagus (recurrent laryngeal branch)
Posterior cricoarytenoid	Abducts the vocal folds	Vagus (recurrent laryngeal branch
Interarytenoids	Adducts the vocal folds	Vagus (both superior and recurrent laryngeal branch)

Innervation of the phonatory system

Four cranial nerves – the vagus (CN10), the trigeminal (CN5), the facial (CN7) and the hypoglossal (CN12) – innervate the muscles of the phonatory system. The vagus nerve is entirely responsible for innervating the intrinsic muscles of the larynx, while CN5, 7 and 12 innervate the extrinsic laryngeal muscles. The following offers a brief guide.

The vagus nerve, which arises from the nucleus ambiguus, divides into three branches, namely:

- the pharyngeal nerve branch, which supplies motor nerve fibres to the pharynx and all the muscles of the soft palate apart from the tensor veli palatini;
- the superior laryngeal nerve branch, which further divides into two parts: the internal laryngeal nerve branch which carries sensory information from the mucous membranes of the epiglottis and the interior of the larynx, and the external laryngeal nerve branch, a motor nerve to the cricothyroid muscle and the inferior pharyngeal constrictor muscle;
- the recurrent laryngeal nerve branch, which innervates all intrinsic muscles of the larynx apart from the cricothyroid muscle (see above).

The trigeminal nerve (CN5) provides a motor nerve supply to the mylohyoid muscle and the anterior belly of the digastricus. The facial nerve (CN7) activates the posterior belly of the digastricus muscle and the stylohyoid muscle. The hypoglossal nerve (CN12) provides a motor nerve supply to the following extrinsic laryngeal muscles: geniohyoid, sternohyoid, omohyoid, thyrohyoid and sternothyroid.

Sensory functions of the larynx

Afferent pathways in the larynx are as important as efferent pathways in terms of phonation, respiration and swallowing. A variety of sensory or proprioceptive receptors are found in considerable numbers in the mucosa of the larynx and in muscles, joints and ligaments, as well as in the lip, tongue and velopharyngeal area. The receptors are involved in both conscious and unconscious tasks involving laryngeal motor skills (Boehme and Gross, 2005). As well as chemoreceptors there exists evidence of various mechanoreceptors. The greatest number of mechanoreceptors appear to be located on the laryngeal surface of the epiglottis with a lower density on the vocal folds (Mathieson, 2001). Rapidly adapting mechanoreceptors within the laryngeal mucosa provide the central nervous system (CNS) with perceptual and proprioceptive afference for voice sound production and airway protection. During any proprioceptal activity the CNS uses all available neural information to choreograph laryngeal activity such as phonation, respiration and swallowing. Hammer and Kruegar (2014) raised the interesting question as to why mechanosensory information, which yields a defensive response when an individual breathes, goes largely unnoticed when an individual phonates. They asked, is there a voice-related modulation of laryngeal mechanosensory detection? Such modulation would be consistent with current models of afferent laryngeal control and in their study they found that the laryngeal sensorium may modulate mechanosensory afference to attenuate the potential distracting influence of sensory input during voice. In addition they noted a difference in men and women during voice tasks, with the latter maintaining a greater sensitivity during the voice task than men, thus causing them to consider whether this might have important implications for the higher prevalence of sensori-motor voice disturbances in women. They also suggest that the healthy larynx exhibits voice-related elevation of mechanosensory detection thresholds and that women may maintain a greater sensitivity (lower thresholds) than men with implications for laryngeal control and maintenance of fluent voice production.

The proprioceptive system, depth and kinaesthetic sensitivity allow control of the actual position of the larynx within the entire vocal and speech system.

The vocal folds

As the thyroarytenoid muscle comprises the bulk of the vocal folds it is important to look at the structure and histology of the vocal folds in more detail. The vocal folds consist of five different layers as follows:

- The outer layer or integument, which maintains the shape of the vocal fold, consists mainly of columnar epithelium apart from the medial edge and is subject to the greatest impact stress of phonation. It is covered by stratified squamous epithelium, thus making this topmost layer much stiffer than the middle layer.
- The middle layer or lamina propria, comprising three layers of connective tissue:
    1. superficial (known as Reinke's space) – consists of pliable, loose, fibrous connections;
    2. intermediate – consists primarily of elastic fibres;
    3. deep – consists of collagen fibres.
- The body or vocalis muscle, which can thicken, shorten and stiffen the vocal folds.

Each layer exhibits varying mechanical properties and is of a different thickness. The relationship between all five will alter significantly, depending on the manner of vibration and the coupling between all the layers (Sato and Hirano, 1997; Mathieson, 2001). Muscle fibres exhibit different mechanical characteristics when they are contracted, in the process of being contracted, or at rest. Similarly, with the variation in the five layers, the mechanical characteristics of the body vary, depending on the amount of heat generated, the variations due to oxygen consumption, blood flow and the amount and type of fibres present – for example, whether these are collagenous or elastic fibres.

In a position superior and lateral to the true vocal folds are the false or ventricular folds, which generally do not vibrate in normal voice production but approximate during swallowing to form a firm preventative seal. In certain conditions, the ventricular folds may adduct to varying degrees and cover the view of the true vocal folds. They are rarely seen to vibrate under examination.

The space between the ventricular and true vocal folds is known as the laryngeal ventricle and it is well supplied with mucous glands, thereby providing lubrication for the vocal folds as a protection in part from the effects of friction.

The resonatory system

The resonatory system consists of the chest, the pharyngeal, oral and nasal cavities and the soft palate. The resonant characteristics of the voice are affected by postural adjustments of the tongue, jaw and lips, as well as through movement of the base of the tongue and the soft palate. The latter is responsible for the addition or subtraction of nasal resonance during speech.

The resonators above the larynx can alter in size, shape and tension with further additional modification occurring through contraction of the pharyngeal and extrinsic laryngeal muscles. While the larynx is, of course, the primary contributor to the production of voice, without the influence of the resonators the voice would lack recognisable characteristics and sound very thin indeed. Speech resonance is the result of the transfer of sound produced by the vocal folds through the vocal tract comprised as has been said of the pharynx, the oral cavity and the nasal cavity (Kummer, 2020; Peterson-Falzone *et al.*, 2017). The vocal tract filters this sound, selectively enhancing harmonics based on the size and/or shape of the vocal tract. Perceived resonance is the result of this filtered tone.

While the velopharyngeal (VP) valve plays an integral role in determining speech resonance, other aspects of the vocal tract also contribute to the perceived sound. These include the size and shape of the resonating cavities, the pharynx, oral cavity, and nasal cavity, the position of the tongue, and the degree of mouth opening.

The pharynx has two muscular layers. The outer layer, which forms the major part of the pharynx, is formed by three pairs of constrictor muscles – the superior, middle and inferior constrictors. These muscles, whose fibres have a circular direction, form the posterior and lateral walls of the pharynx, while the anterior portion of the pharynx affords a linkage to the nasal, oral and laryngeal sections of the pharynx. These 'linkages' are known, respectively, as the nasopharynx, oropharynx and laryngopharynx. The constrictor muscles function, as the name suggests, to constrict the pharynx during swallowing or gagging. The inner muscular layer of the pharynx, which forms the pharyngeal tube, is composed of the stylopharyngeus, salpingopharyngeus and palatopharyngeus muscles, whose fibres have a longitudinal direction, which contract to lift the pharynx during swallowing. In addition, contraction of the palatopharyngeus narrows the Pillars of Fauces, the archway between the pharyngeal and oral cavities which is formed by the tongue, anterior and posterior tonsillar pillars, and soft palate. Contraction of the stylopharyngeus helps to move the lateral walls of the pharynx medially.

Resonance is the amplification or reinforcement of vibration, normally by a hollow cavity or space (Bunch Dayme, 2005). Resonatory chambers have different characteristics and their effect on the voice changes due to the size, shape, type of opening, composition and thickness of the walls, surface and combinations of the above. As a brief, general statement regarding the effect of resonance on vocal quality, the shape and flexibility of the resonating chamber determines which frequencies are enhanced. Larger resonators respond most to low frequencies, while resonating chambers which are rigid experience the least damping. Resonators that are flexible and mobile tend to incur greater damping but are more universal in enhancement.

Innervation of the resonatory system

Branches of several different cranial nerves are responsible for the innervation of the muscles of the resonatory system. Motor supply for the two muscular layers of the pharynx is innervated by cranial nerves CN9, CN10 and CN11, collectively termed the pharyngeal plexus. Sensory information from the pharynx, the Pillars of Fauces and from four of the five muscle pairs that form the soft palate is sent by CN7 and the sensory branch of CN9. Motor innervation for the soft palate, apart from the tensor palatini which is innervated by the mandibular branch of CN5, the trigeminal, is from the spinal accessory nerve or CN11.

The function and innervation of the muscles of the resonatory system are given in Table 1.6.

Posture and alignment

Voice is the result of a combined effort by all three of the systems discussed above, respiratory, phonatory and resonatory. What must be remembered, however, is that these systems

Table 1.6 Muscles of the resonatory system

Muscle	Function	Innervation
Inferior constrictor	Constricts the pharynx	Spinal accessory nerve and laryngeal branch of vagus
Medial and superior constrictors	Constricts the pharynx	Spinal accessory
Palatopharyngeus	Raises the pharynx, narrows the Pillars of Fauces, lowers the soft palate	Spinal accessory
Salpingopharyngeus	Raises the pharynx	Spinal accessory
Stylopharyngeus	Raises the pharynx and helps in medial movement of pharyngeal walls	Glossopharyngeal
Levator palatini	Raises the soft palate	Spinal accessory
Palatoglossus	Lowers the soft palate	Spinal accessory
Uvulus	Shortens the soft palate	Spinal accessory
Tensor palatini	Tenses the soft palate	Trigeminal

are directly affected by posture. In turn, posture is affected by the movement of the bony skeleton and the muscles and tendons that support it. Virtually every bone in the body is connected to another bone through bone/muscle connection. Most muscles are attached to bones by connecting tendon, thick, tough cords of tissue that connect bone and muscle. Tendons grow directly out of muscle fibre and connect to the outer layer of the associated bone. Many bones have protrusions where the tendon connects which provide extra surface area for a secure join. Tendons are strong enough to withstand tension when muscles contract to move the bone, the tendon acts as a space-saving 'connector' that transfers the movement of the muscle to the bone; each muscle attaches to two bones and the push and pull of the muscle moves the bones in relationship to each other.

The intimate connection of muscle, tendon and bone allows freedom of movement, but it also means that movement of one body part will affect another and so the intimate inter-relationship of head, neck and back, the positioning of the spine and pelvis will affect the ribcage and consequently respiration and phonation.

The ageing process

Although the anatomy and physiology of the larynx is well documented, individual differences and variability should be recognised. Empirical data on the larynx continue to be collected and information is continually updated, with any consensus on the 'norm' being open to revision as empirical research is ongoing. As more information is gained so there may be changes to what is considered empirical evidence. It is, however, safe to say that our current knowledge supports the view that many factors influence the changes in voice that occur throughout life from changes in the volume and shape of the vocal tract and rib cage, through to the biochemical histological morphology of the vocal fold. In terms of our current knowledge of normal development and ageing the following changes from birth through to older age occur.

In the infant, the larynx is high in the vocal tract at birth, with the lower border of the cricoid cartilage at a level between cervical vertebrae 3 and 4 (C3-C4), which allows the infant to alternate rapidly between sucking and breathing simultaneously without aspirating. The protection of the airway is further enhanced by the ary-epiglottic folds by their thickness and by the introversion of the epiglottis to the glottis level of the arytenoids. The hyoid bone and thyroid cartilage function as one and the opening to the larynx is narrow due to the shape of the cartilages in infancy. As well as differences in the cartilages, the vocal fold structure in newborns and children is much less refined, and the vocal fold mucosa is thinner in newborns and young children, with a high percentage of collagen and no discernible difference between the layers of lamina propria, rather like that of Reinke's space in adults. The infant vocal fold is deficient in the anterior and posterior macula flava fibres, which in turn leads to less anchoring strength to the laryngeal architecture. At birth the membranous portion of the vocal fold accounts for 50% of the total fold length. As the child matures the membranous portion lengthens relative to the arytenoids. The different layers in the structure are not clearly seen in newborns and young children and first appear between 1 and 4 years, after which they are clearly visible. The vocal folds are between 2.5 and 3.0 mm in length (Mathieson, 2001; Scott Howard and Berke, 2012). By 5 years old vocal fold length has increased to approximately 7.5 mm, with this gradual increase in vocal fold length continuing until puberty. Hormonal changes in male and female larynges, due to increased oestrogen secretions in the female and increased androgen secretions in the male, herald a notable change in the size of the larynx and the length of the vocal folds. By this age the larynx has moved lower in the vocal tract to a level between cervical vertebrae 6 and 7 (C6-C7).

The greatest change is noted in the male larynx, where the angle of the thyroid decreases from 120 to 90 degrees, contributing to the much more visible laryngeal outline in the male. The female larynx by contrast shows much less dramatic change at puberty than that of the male. The angle of the thyroid cartilage does not change significantly and although the larynx and vocal tract increase in size the effect on overall pitch and resonance is much more limited. Titze (1994a) suggests that at this age, the length of female vocal folds is approximately 12–17 mm, while those of the male may be between 17 and 23 mm. As a consequence of this increase in length there is a fairly dramatic drop in the fundamental frequency of the male voice, often by one octave. Average speaking fundamental frequencies are generally considered to be 128 Hz in men and 225 Hz in women, with graduated changes through the range in ascending order from low to high related to vocal classification: bass, baritone, tenor for men and contralto, mezzo-soprano, soprano for women. Interesting work on the fundamental frequency of the voice as a highly dimorphic trait indicates that in women, voice attractiveness is correlated with facial attractiveness, higher-pitched voices are rated as more attractive and more juvenile than lower-pitched voices. Females would seem to prefer male voices with lowered fundamental frequencies to those with raised fundamental frequencies. Women prefer deeper male voices (Collins, 2000; Puts *et al.*, 2007).

Hirano and Kurita (1986) suggest that full vocal ligaments have been developed for both male and females by age 15, while Mathieson (2001) notes that the mutational period of the singing voice lasts much longer than the mutational period of the speaking voice, so it is important to be aware of vocal vulnerability at this time.

Changes in vocal quality as a feature of ageing may occur for a variety of reasons throughout adulthood. In some cases these are gender-specific, for example, as a result of female hormonal change at puberty, during pregnancy and pre-, during and post-menopause. Temporary changes (except at the menopause) may be the result of a number of factors such as a decrease in oestrogen, water retention, oedema, venous dilation of vocal fold tissue and increased vocal fold mass. Conversely, no statistically significant changes were reported in the following studies into the effect of the hormonal cycle on the singer's voice (Ryan and Kenny, 2009); the influence of the menstrual cycle on voice and speech in adolescents (Meurer *et al.*, 2009); or voice onset time as a function of oral contraceptive use (Morris *et al.*, 2009), although change was reported by some subjects anecdotally. Hamdan *et al.* (2009) concluded that pregnancy has limited effect on the speaking voice; vocal symptoms in pregnant women versus controls showed no significant differences in their study, although vocal fatigue was more prevalent in the pregnant group. They noted that with respect to the acoustic parameters there was significant decrease in the maximum phonation time (MPT) at term but this increased significantly post-delivery. Any changes noted throughout pregnancy were considered to be an artefact of the physiological, anatomical and metabolic adaptations that occur during gestation. Possible permanent changes at the menopause can be not only as a result of all of the above but also the result of tissue structure changes within the folds that relate to the physiology of ageing and are therefore non-gender-specific. These changes may include alteration to the vocal fold cover, epithelial thickening changes in the underlying connective tissue which result in looser linkage of the epithelium to the deeper tissues. The elastic fibres of the vocal ligament break down and become thinner while the mucous glands degenerate, resulting in less adequate lubrication of the vocal fold surface and probable changes in the biomechanical properties of the superficial epithelium. As with other muscles, the laryngeal muscles are prone to atrophy, which means that there are fewer muscle fibres in each muscle. In addition, the surviving fibres tend to be thinner and to show significant degenerative changes. It is possible that these changes result from disturbances of the blood supply. Joint suppleness is affected by a loss of collagen fibres and by degeneration. Cartilages progressively harden and begin to ossify and calcify, although this change tends to be slower in females. Abitbol (2006) suggests that the anterior part of the arytenoid cartilage, the point of insertion for the vocal fold and the epiglottic cartilage, does not ossify but loses elasticity. Pleural, oral, nasal and vocal tract tissue is thinner and drier.

As a result of the reduction in bulk, muscle tone and elasticity there is often a noticeable rise in male fundamental frequency with increasing age. Female atrophic changes tend to be less significant, but the reduction of ovarian hormones at the menopause often increases oedema in the superficial layer of the lamina propria, with a concomitant change in the bulk of the vocal folds leading to a lower fundamental frequency. The impact of hormone replacement therapy on menopausal women has been studied in some detail (D'haeseleer *et al.*, 2009, 2011). Study findings suggest that menopause lowers the speaking fundamental frequency by approximately 14 Hz, but that this decrease is counteracted by hormone replacement therapy. Their work opines that post-menopausal women with and without hormone therapy possess good vocal quality overall. They suggest that in post-menopausal women without hormone therapy, body mass index should be taken into account, as body mass index is positively correlated to the speaking fundamental frequency in this group. Their study results would appear to highlight some difference of opinion between researchers as to whether female voice quality deteriorates after natural or surgically induced menopause (Caruso *et al.*, 2000; Amir *et al.*, 2003; Amir and Biron-Shental, 2004; Firat *et al.*, 2009; Yezdan *et al.*, 2009).

The importance of hyaluronic acid (HA) in maintenance of the vocal fold structure and function along with the impact on the ageing process of the male and female voice has produced interesting data; for example:

- the influence of HA on the biomechanical properties of the vocal fold cover and its likely contribution to the maintenance of an optimal tissue viscosity (Chan *et al.*, 2001);

- the key role of HA in tissue viscosity, shock absorption and space filling with particular reference to the larynx and voice (Ward *et al.*, 2002);
- gender-related differences in HA distribution in the human vocal fold and the implication of less protection from phonotrauma for the female vocal folds (Butler *et al.*, 2001);
- the viscoelasticity of HA and its use in lamina propria replacement therapy where, due to vocal fold scarring, the lamina propria is lost or deficient (Chhetri and Mendelsohn, 2010; Hirano *et al.*, 2009).

The impact of changes in the histological biomechanical morphology of the vocal fold play a critical role in the ageing voice; for example:

- age-related alterations in the deposition of extracellular matrix (ECM) have been reported by Ohno *et al.* (2009);
- age-related changes of collagenous fibres in vocal fold mucosa including excessive accumulation of collagen, dense collagen bundles, reduced elastin and decreased HA (Sato *et al.*, 2002);
- the activity of the fibroblasts in the maculae flavae decreases and less HA is produced (Bruzzi *et al.*, 2017);
- a slowdown in collagen turnover with ageing may increase the cross-linking of collagen molecules, which in turn may explain in part the stiffness in the vocal folds that occur with age (Ding and Gray, 2001).

As well as the changes in the larynx, ageing brings about neurological, physiological and skeletal change. These changes may include reduced efficiency of the control systems, such as reduced efficiency of neural transmission to initiate laryngeal movement resulting in, for example, impaired vocal fold approximation, which leads to reduced glottal efficiency. The sensitivity of the airway is reduced and the 'repel' mechanism is less frequently triggered. With increasing age, reduction in the mobility of the ribcage occurs; the ribs become less mobile and respiratory function may become compromised. As Mathieson (2001) notes, by the age of 75 respiratory efficiency is half that of a 30-year-old. Declining respiratory function will, of course, affect vocal quality, as there is a loss of breath support for voicing. Although even healthy older adults are likely to undergo reduced physiological function due to changes to the laryngeal and respiratory musculature, Maslan *et al.* (2011) suggest that in healthy older adults (65 years and older) without debilitating comorbidities, MPT can approach the durations seen in young adults. This is somewhat different to the results of the relatively few studies undertaken on MPT in older adults. Across all age groups, men on average have been considered to be able to sustain a longer MPT than women, but this gender difference was not notable in that it was not statistically different in the Maslan study. This widens the spectrum of what should be considered normal in older adults without significant health problems or underlying laryngeal pathology. Many of the individuals in their cohort could phonate for 20 seconds in the absence of pathology. Another aspect of ageing which should be considered is that of loss of teeth, which causes the upper and lower lips to lose support, and as a consequence of the loss of teeth the jaw decalcifies and erodes. Abitbol (2006) notes that paradoxically, lack of teeth means the mouth is no longer able to open fully and the joint of the jaw therefore becomes less supple. Mouth opening is of course essential for articulatory precision and for additional oral resonance to the voice.

It should, however, be remembered that the process and effects of ageing are very arbitrary. Circumstantial factors that can influence ageing include lifestyle choices, smoking, alcohol abuse, diet, environmental or workplace factors such as dust or chemical vapours, certain digestive diseases such as gastroesophageal reflux or pharyngolaryngeal reflux. As already noted, for some individuals ageing does not equal vocal deterioration because their maintenance of respiratory function and mobility assures vocal quality. For others, however, ageing may bring limited mobility, multiple medications and lack of motivation or opportunity to communicate, so leading to an increasing decline in vocal quality and communicative efficacy and efficiency. Key to maintaining and preserving vocal power and vocal efficiency is to consider aspects over which the individual has control, such as physical exercise, hydration, dental care and diet. Aspects over which the individual has less control, such as reduced hearing acuity, should also be considered. Hearing acuity reduces with age and presbycusis is known to occur in over half of all people over 60 years (Deafness Research UK, www.deafnessresearch.org.uk). Auditory feedback is of course an essential tool in monitoring and controlling vocal quality and, for an older person, in preserving and enhancing communication channels.

It is important to remember the impact on an older person of reduced communication opportunities and the ability to make the most of such. Age UK's Loneliness and Isolation Evidence Review of 2015 reported that over one million people say they always or often feel lonely and 49% of all people aged 75 and over live alone. Indeed, it has been recognised for many years that older people may experience isolation and loneliness, which may be compounded by a reduction in adequacy of communication caused by voice weakness or disorder and which may have a huge impact on quality of life. Attendance at a social group may be one of few weekly contacts outside the home environment, creating a source of cognitive, emotional and social stimulation, maintaining interest in others and contributing to self-esteem within the community. For those reasons, even a minor improvement in voice quality and limitation of further deterioration is vital for the older person and their communication status. If optimal voice is achieved, then communication opportunities can be maximised and quality of life enhanced. Older people should never become a lower priority on the caseload simply due to age. On the contrary, a small number of clinical contact hours may well improve the patient's situation considerably with a parallel improvement in quality of life.

Organisations such as The Silver Line Helpline was set up in the UK to offer a confidential helpline to combat loneliness in the older population; in 2019 it joined with Age UK in this initiative. The Jo Cox Commission on Loneliness reported in 2017, highlighting the issue of loneliness in the UK and The Jo Cox Foundation has also joined with Age UK to try and alter the lives of older lonely people in the UK. Undoubtedly other countries will have similar initiatives.

Summary

As an advocate of a knowledge-based problem-solving approach as the foundation of clinical assessment and intervention when working with voice disorders, the author is of the firm opinion that this approach is only possible if it is based on sound knowledge and a critical appraisal of the constellation of factors that affect the patient and thus their voice.

Understanding voice disorders must begin with an understanding of 'the normal'. It is only through knowledge and understanding of normal anatomy, physiology, neuroanatomy and neurophysiology of 'voice' that a differential diagnosis is possible.

In offering a brief, easily accessible overview of the structures and functions central to the production of voice, noting how they change over time; in examining the influence of life events, lifestyle choice and ageing on the voice will, it is hoped, better inform the clinical process of reaching a differential diagnosis. A process which must, of course, be done in partnership with the patient.

2

THE SPECTRUM OF VOICE
DISORDERS - CLASSIFICATION

Introduction

There have been many approaches to the classification of voice disorders over the years, with experts attempting to find agreement on the best system of classification. Undoubtedly, a unified classification would be extremely beneficial to all involved as the variety of terms can create confusion and lead to difficulty in making useful comparisons, not only for research purposes but for clinical discussion. For example, some use the terms 'functional' and 'psychogenic' interchangeably, while others make clear distinction between these terms. Similarly, the terms 'organic' and 'non-organic' were once widely used to describe voice disorders, but these terms are by their nature somewhat non-specific, although they make a useful differentiation between those disorders which are the result of pathological changes to the vocal folds and those which are not. It should, however, be noted that, even within the overarching term of non-organic voice disorders, the term is slightly ambiguous, as some patterns of misuse can lead to organic changes.

Clearly, there are advantages and disadvantages in most classification systems, but there are few patients who present with a 'classic' voice disorder which fits neatly into a single category. Indeed, many disorders 'overlap', have secondary presentations and have contributions from more than one aetiologic factor (Stemple *et al.*, 2013). Voice disorders are not mutually exclusive and overlap is common as in, for example, the aetiology of nodules. Nodules result from vocal misuse, a functional cause, but the vocal misuse results in repeated trauma to the vocal folds which may then lead to structural changes to the vocal folds.

As with most evolving disciplines, so too with voice disorders and while there are a number of new and emerging classification systems, the author has selected that of Baker *et al.* (2007), the diagnostic classification system for voice disorders (DCSVD), which makes a distinction between Organic Voice Disorder (OVD) and Functional Voice Disorder (FVD), with Psychogenic Voice Disorder and Muscle Tension Dysphonia as subtypes of FVD. Further subtypes of OVD, PVD and FVD were also detailed, leading to a full classification system. For the purposes of this book the DCSVD terminology forms a broad guide for discussion of voice disorders with the following sections:

- Functional Voice Disorder – Muscle Tension Dysphonia: this disorder involves a structurally normal larynx which is subject to muscle dysfunction, although all disorders do not demonstrate the same patterns of muscle tension.
- Functional Voice Disorder – Psychogenic: this disorder involves a structurally normal larynx which is subject to psychological stressors leading to habitual, maladaptive aphonia or dysphonia.

- Organic Voice Disorder – Structural: this disorder results from tissue change or trauma to the larynx.
- Organic Voice Disorder – Neurogenic: this disorder results from damage to, or disorder in, the central or peripheral nervous system innervations to the larynx.

The choice of a classification system may well be determined by the clinician's place of work and working practice. This chapter will explore the spectrum of voice disorders, while Chapter 3 offers practical descriptions of those disorders most commonly found on clinical caseloads.

There are several other disorders which, despite different views as to the appropriateness of referral, are part of the referral experience of many clinicians and form discrete and unique groups. For this reason they will be discussed later in the chapter so that the specific challenges and issues can be explored. These topics are: Professional and Occupational Voice Users, Gender Dysphoria, Inducible Laryngeal Obstruction, Chronic Cough and Aerophagia.

Functional voice disorders

Muscle tension dysphonia

Into this section of the Functional Voice Disorder classification fall disorders that involve poor muscle function or misuse, which may or may not lead to secondary pathology. However, vocal misuse and hyperfunction are often the cause of tissue changes to the vocal folds, which give rise to lesions such as nodules and polyps and may be contributing factors in some organic conditions, along with lifestyle choices such as smoking or alcohol intake. In reality there is often a sequence of events, which may be the catalyst to the eventual Muscle Tension Dysphonia. Irritation to the delicate mucosal linings of the pharynx or larynx can create discomfort, increased production of secretions, coughing and/or throat clearing, muscle misuse and hyperfunction. Discomfort and pain in the throat or neck may be the first symptom noted by the patient in the course of the disorder (Roy *et al.*, 2009).

Irritation to the larynx may also be the result of acute or chronic inflammation, which may be secondary to upper respiratory infection or caused by allergy or the presence of irritants in the environment such as fumes, airborne particles or cigarette smoke. Laryngeal irritation may be caused by acid repeatedly refluxing from the stomach into the oesophagus alone, known as gastroesophageal reflux disease (GORD). However, if the stomach acid travels up the oesophagus and spills into the pharynx and larynx, even on occasion into the back of the nasal airway, leading to inflammation in areas not protected against gastric acid exposure, such as the vocal folds, it is known as laryngopharyngeal reflux (LPR). With LPR, you may not have the classic symptoms of GORD, such as a burning sensation in your lower chest (heartburn). That's why it can be difficult to diagnose and why it is often called 'silent reflux'. Both LPR and GORD are frequently described as the cause of laryngeal irritation and proton pump inhibitors (PPIs) prescribed to treat the GORD/LPR. Khidr *et al.* (2003) report significant reduction in hoarseness and throat clearing after two months of such treatment, which reinforces the view that if the root of the irritation is correctly diagnosed and treated, the problem may resolve spontaneously and relatively quickly. However, there still remains some ambivalence about the side effects of long-term PPI use (*British Medical Journal*, 2012; Ambizas and Etzel, 2017).

Whatever the cause of the vocal tract irritation, the latter is often the precursor to the development of MTD. As the patient experiences discomfort and increased secretion production, it is almost inevitable that throat clearing and frequent/sometimes excessive coughing may result. This may lead to increased irritation to the delicate mucosa, disturbance to voice production, voice quality and the health of the laryngeal tissues. The resulting voice quality is generally hoarse, husky, breathy or low-pitched. Whatever the term used, trauma to the laryngeal tissue, which results in voice quality change, can be the result of one isolated episode of vocal misuse but, more usually, is the result of extended periods of vocal misuse or trauma.

The following are some common examples of causative factors:

Yelling, screaming and shouting. These are all instances where voice is produced by hyperadduction with increased tension of the vocal folds. While pathological changes generally occur after prolonged misuse, an afternoon shouting at a sports match or an evening of karaoke may equally result in laryngeal oedema. Karaoke bars are a very popular form of entertainment and present multiple opportunities for vocal misuse.

Frequent use of hard glottal attack. This is a manner of initiating vowels in which the vocal folds adduct rapidly and completely, building up subglottic air pressure until it is released as an abrupt explosion to initiate phonation. It is frequently a predisposing factor in vocal fold trauma.

Throat clearing and coughing. These are often presenting symptoms of vocal misuse. Patients may be unaware that they are coughing frequently, or else may complain of a 'frog' or 'tickle' that needs to be eliminated by clearing the throat. When the vocal folds are irritated by these activities they become bathed in mucous in an effort to reduce friction. Patients often perpetuate the problem by trying to get rid of this lubrication by again clearing the throat.

Irritants such as smoking, alcohol and environmental pollution. These can result in a 'dry throat'. The laryngeal mucosa becomes very dry and the vocal folds are more prone to damage. Birth control pills, antihistamines, and some prescription medication such as inhaled corticosteroids (ICS), for example those used by asthmatics, may also have a drying effect on the laryngeal mucosa. Vocal problems as side effects of inhaled corticosteroids in asthma patients have been the subject of a number of studies (Buhl, 2006; Simberg *et al.*, 2009). Bhalla *et al.* (2009) measured laryngeal function in regular ICS users and found that regular ICS users were significantly more likely to have abnormal jitter, shimmer and closed-phase quotient scores. They reported on local side effects which can include pain, chronic sore throat, habitual throat clearing and laryngeal irritation with subsequent dysphonia. Saeed *et al.* (2018) reported on impaired voice quality and various grades of dysphonia in patients with COPD and bronchial asthma in relation to disease severity and medication, noting that acoustic analysis showed a highly significant increase in jitter and shimmer and decreased harmonic-to-noise ratio in 100% of patients of both groups. They concluded that all COPD and bronchial asthma patients had dysphonia, either due to organic causes or due to functional causes. Voice changes were directly correlated with degree of severity and fluticasone propionate inhalation use in bronchial asthma patients, and with ipratropium bromide inhalation in the COPD group. These studies contrast with that of Kim *et al.* (2011), who found no significant changes associated with dysphonia, either in the perceptual or acoustic studies of asthmatics.

Singing with inadequate vocal technique or in poor environmental conditions. Into this group falls the amateur or semi-professional singer who has limited voice training and who is working in clubs or venues where there is inadequate ventilation. Under these conditions there is often excessive demand placed on the voice, as the individual may have to sing over the sound of highly amplified musical instruments. Channels such as YouTube, where individuals post self-recorded performances, may also compound vocal misuse.

Talking against a high level of background noise. This is often necessary for occupational or social reasons. As a result of the desire to be heard, people often raise the volume of their voices and, due to the increased laryngeal tension, vocal fold trauma and irritation are likely to occur.

Extended periods of voice use. Work on the physiology of voice (Titze *et al.*, 2007; Hunter and Titze, 2009) has identified the need to counteract the damaging effect of vocal loading with periods of respite. While it is possible to talk intermittently for long periods, there are limits to every larynx and some larynges are more vulnerable than others.

Conversely, some patients may have even severe dysphonia due to MTD but no secondary pathology. Suffice it to say that, whether the MTD results in secondary pathology or not, the aetiology of the voice disorder provides many keys to treatment and management. As Mathieson (2001) noted, 'many of the vocal symptoms of psychogenic voice disorders are similar to those patients with muscle tension dysphonia. The voice is frequently effortful to produce and the patient describes vocal fatigue and in many instances vocal tract discomfort'.

While the voice problem may manifest as musculoskeletal tension and hyperkinetic behaviours, it is interesting to note that in the wider functional group (FVD), which includes MTD, there is now an acknowledgement that many of the aetiological features of psychogenic voice disorder are also to be found within this population. What is certain is that the treatment of medically unexplained symptoms in Ear, Nose and Throat has changed in recent years; there is now more emphasis on psychological factors due to an association with anxiety and depression (Ullas *et al.*, 2013). Kolbrunner and Seifert (2015) said 'Clinicians believe that psychosocial factors play a causal role in the aetiology of many forms of functional dysphonia (FD). But for decades all attempts to confirm such causation have failed'. The authors contend that the reason for that is due to the focus on evidence-based medicine, where outcome measures are by their very nature quantitative, in contrast to the appraisal and evaluation of therapy which by its nature is often qualitative. It is hoped that in the future there may be more opportunities to privilege qualitative research in the identification of the causal role played by psychosocial factors in the aetiology of functional dysphonia. The need to consider the inclusion of a psychosocial interview as part of every case history interview when working with patients with voice disorders is further developed in Chapter 4.

Psychogenic voice disorder

Given the acknowledgement above that many aetiological features of psychogenic voice disorders are also found in MTD, to separate the sections may seem artificial but, in the author's opinion, justified, in that psychogenic voice disorder describes a non-organic voice disorder where there is no structural or neurological pathology to account for the disordered vocal quality as the vocal folds are essentially normal in structure and movement and the aetiology is psychological in origin. Baker *et al.* (2007) suggest that a psychogenic disturbance 'occurs in the absence of structural or neurological pathology sufficient to account for the voice difficulty, with onset and maintenance of the voice difficulty caused by disturbed psychological processes'. The work of Butcher *et al.* (2007) and their development of a model for understanding and treating psychogenic voice disorders using a cognitive behavioural therapy (CBT) framework is to be recommended and acknowledged. This model applies the concept of a psychological conversion disorder to voice disorders with a clear psychogenic aetiology. It distinguishes between two types of conversion, one that is likely to be intractable to any type of therapy and the other, more common type that can be responsive to the psychological interventions of CBT, combined with appropriate amounts of physiological voice therapy. This classification model distinguishes psychogenic conversion voice disorders from muscle tension disorders. It does, however, acknowledge that muscle tension voice disorders, whilst not conversion disorders, may well have a degree of stress contributing to the onset and maintenance of the voice problem. Their model has implications for assessment and for treatment. It requires careful exploration of the psychological features in the case history to be able to arrive at a confident diagnosis and it requires a level of psychological therapy to be sensitively matched to these features.

The early symptoms of some disorders such as myasthenia gravis, Parkinson's disease, multiple sclerosis or even carcinoma have the possibility of a misdiagnosis of psychogenic dysphonia. It is therefore critical that although many patients may present with what appear to be classic symptoms of psychogenic dysphonia, this diagnosis should not be made lightly and a diagnosis should be reached after exclusion of laryngeal pathology through detailed and thorough examination, such as videostroboscopic and stroboscopic examination, and only when thorough assessment has been completed and other possibilities excluded should the clinician arrive at a diagnosis of psychogenic dysphonia.

In psychogenic dysphonia, the vocal folds under layngoscopic examination are of normal appearance, are capable of adduction, move normally and adequately yet presentation is inconsistent, in that a normal note might be heard on vegetative and reflexive functions, such as coughing, laughing, sneezing, yawning, throat clearing and occasionally even intermittently for phonation, yet this is unpredictable on purposeful phonation. The vocal folds may be seen to approximate initially or intermittently but will quickly abduct so that phonation is inhibited. Air may flow between the vocal folds with little resistance so that phonation length is short and any attempted voice is breathy or intermittent. In some patients communication may be produced by 'mouthing' speech with complete cessation of outgoing airflow with glottal closure to block the out breath, or normal tidal breathing may continue throughout the communication, with no coordination with the spoken words. In other patients, there may be cessation of outgoing airflow and the production of ejectives while breath is held or even voice produced on an ingressive air stream. Surprisingly, in some of these patients, there appears to be little discomfort associated with these very disordered patterns of respiration for speech. When phonation is attempted, the vocal quality may vary greatly from mild breathiness to severe forced and effortful voice or total aphonia. The disorder may present with a constant disturbance to voice production or be intermittent, involving the transition from consonant to vowels or momentary loss of phonation on certain syllables of words only, or on entire words or phrases. The intermittent aphonia or dysphonia may be in evidence and related to the subject matter being discussed or be apparently random. The disturbance may be of pitch or volume at a consistently inappropriate level or may be heard as sudden pitch breaks or sudden change in volume of voice.

In some patients it can be incongruous that such a disabling disorder can be so readily accepted with various life changes made by the patient and significant others. In case discussions, clinicians will often report patients who have lived for years with bizarre arrangements within the family to accommodate their aphonia and with an apparent ease and acceptance that is out of line with the major changes being undertaken (Mathieson, 2001). Similarly, patients may assert that the situation 'is fine' and poses no real difficulties, appearing oblivious to the unusual arrangements they are accepting. Some patients, however, may give strong assurances of high motivation towards a resolution, but with little active cooperation or acknowledgement of success in any therapy. Others may project blame on to various professionals who have been involved with them to date for misdiagnosis or failure to diagnose, thus justifying the continuing dysphonia.

Initial discussion should underline the fact that no structural abnormalities or disease exists within the larynx to account for the vocal symptoms and should highlight the patient's ability to achieve voice again within the therapy session. Treatment should begin with a simple explanation of how voice is produced, underlining the fact that the patient has the mechanical capacity to achieve vocal fold adduction, but that currently this is not occurring. As a preliminary step, release of tension and breathing exercises may be carried out. The patient should be gently encouraged to achieve voice through vegetative functions, such as a cough or a laugh or indeed on a yawn, a sigh or a hum. It should be noted that sneezing, coughing and laughing may also produce normal voice. Success in producing voice with one of these methods is usually achieved in the first session and once the patient can produce voice by this means, therapy should build on the sound obtained. This may be done by shaping the vegetative sound into a vowel, then graduating to nonsense syllables, single words and phrases. Once the patient feels confident that voice is consistent, the clinician should encourage conversational speech, giving continued positive reinforcement and encouragement, so motivating them to keep using voice after leaving the clinic. Ideally a follow-up session should be planned as soon as possible to reinforce the improved voice quality.

While standard voice therapy alone for the management of Psychogenic Voice Disorders (and FVD) has value, it is suggested that there may be greater value in combining voice therapy with psychological therapies; certainly, working psychologically with the voice should be an important part of the therapeutic intervention. More recently Baker (2017) suggests that person-centred and relational and grief counselling should be part of the intervention process alongside standard voice therapy.

In looking at skill acquisition for clinicians working with voice patients, Butcher *et al.* (2007) state that 'All Speech and Language Therapists working in voice should have basic counselling skills and work within a framework of clinical supervision'. They go on to say, 'SLTs should have on-going access to a clinical psychologist or a CBT specialist for the management of complex cases'. Baker (2010) suggests that one way to achieve this is 'to seek regular supervision from experienced voice practitioners and those with advanced credentials in psychotherapy, or to work conjointly with other mental health professionals'.

In looking at future intervention approaches the author strongly supports Baker's (2010) view that 'Postgraduate training in counselling or psychotherapeutic models such as transactional analysis, systems and family therapy, narrative therapy and cognitive behaviour therapies (CBT) are available to health professionals and can be readily integrated with traditional speech-language pathology practices', a view endorsed by Kolbrunner and Seifert (2015).

Miller *et al.* (2014) proposed the view that 'Allied health professionals are increasingly being trained to use CBT skills in the management of a number of symptoms/illnesses, and this should be considered for the management of functional dysphonia'. This proposal is being followed up through a trial training speech therapists in CBT to treat medically unexplained dysphonia (Deary, 2018).

Globus

Many patients report experiencing a feeling of 'having a lump in their throat' and, while an occasional sensation of a lump in the throat is relatively common in the presence of strong emotion, when, for example, trying not to cry or when having to 'swallow one's feelings', true globus is usually experienced persistently. Patients will report discomfort, will try to swallow, cough or clear the throat in order to dislodge this sensation. While globus symptoms may have both psychogenic and physical origins, all patients should undergo careful examination to exclude the presence of disease or malignant tumour. Some possible causes of globus, in addition to stress and anxiety, are pharyngeal inflammatory conditions, GORD, abnormal upper oesophageal sphincter function, rare tumours, thyroid disease or previously lodged objects which were not completely removed. Other possible but relatively rarely documented causes, therefore needing more studies to confirm their findings, are temporo-mandibular joint (TMJ) disorders, an inability to produce enough saliva, cervical osteophytes or bone spurs and Eagle's syndrome. Eagle's syndrome is a condition associated with the elongation of the styloid process or calcification of the stylohyoid ligament, clinically characterised by throat and neck pain, radiating into the ear.

Mathieson (2001) suggests that discussion and support with reassurance concerning the aetiology of the globus symptom is effective in the majority of patients. Some suggestions for therapy are included in Chapter 7, but it should be noted that globus can be difficult to treat, with symptoms lasting for some time and often recurring.

Mutational falsetto/puberphonia

Mutational Falsetto (MF) has been variously described by authors as occurring in a post-adolescent male who continues to have a pre-adolescent voice (Stemple *et al.*, 2013), or as Juvenile Voice, when a post-adolescent female has the vocal qualities of a child. In the case of a post-adolescent male, it is also known as Puberphonia or Persistent Falsetto (Nicolosi *et al.*, 2004).

For the purposes of this section, concentration will be on the young post-adolescent male, as instances of Juvenile Voice are very rare according to Hedge (2001). Normal male adolescent voice changes during puberty, namely register and pitch breaks, generally resolve without problem and an adult male voice is achieved. For some adolescents, however, despite normal laryngeal growth and the development of secondary sexual characteristics, voice mutation fails to occur and the individual retains his pre-pubertal voice. As with any case history-taking it is very important that the clinician accesses information about the patient's voice and vocal behaviour both before and during puberty and in the more recent past.

A psychogenic aetiology is generally ascribed to this disorder, for reasons such as resisting pubertal changes, a dislike of the new pitch after puberty, embarrassment about the newly developing low-pitched voice (Stemple *et al.*, 2013), a mismatch between the new pitch and their personality, or a rejection of the roles and responsibility of adulthood. Cavalli (2016) suggests that the following issues should be investigated: Did the voice break early? Was there any self-consciousness that may have led to inhibition of voice mutation? Was there a rapid growth spurt that coincided with the voice instability? Were there issues related to a history of singing, for example, were there any signs that the individual tried to maintain a treble singing voice?

Hedge (2001) suggests that some patients may identify more with females, while Lim *et al.* (2007) cite anatomical differences as a possible cause. In the absence of any pathophysiology – for example, persistent hyperfunction of the cricothyroid muscles, the backward tilting of the cricoid cartilage so the vocal folds remain in a state of laxity – it must be assumed that the disorder is behavioural and/or psychogenic in origin, although the communication of this to the patient must be carried out with great sensitivity. It is, of course, critical to access the patient's judgement about the relative impact of their voice on daily activities, but for most patients it may be a cause of embarrassment and stigma. There is often distress at the perceived 'failure' to develop a mature voice and social consequences for males about whom value judgements are made regarding maturity and gender. As discussed above, the causes of puberphonia may be traumatic or emotional situations which have remained unresolved or repressed. They may be anxiety-related, a conversion symptom or involve emotional gain for the patient. Based on clinical examination, laryngoscopic and video stroboscopic findings, and acoustic analysis, the clinician may decide, on occasion, that there is a need to discuss onward referral in addition.

Intervention may comprise a number of different approaches with the aim of therapy to achieve a mature male voice. As the larynx will have been held consistently in an elevated position, work on lowering the larynx should be the initial target for voice therapy. Exercises which release tongue tension offer a good starting point, lip trills and lax vox exercises are recommended. Direct vocal manipulation is recommended by Stemple *et al.* (2013) in order for the patient to experience the new pitch and then to hear the difference between their habitual pitch and the new lower pitch. Vocal manipulation and compression of the larynx has been described by authors such as Lim *et al.* (2007), who suggest pressing downward with the fingers on the thyroid cartilage to hold the larynx down and prevent it from moving upward during phonation. Dagli *et al.* (2008) suggest downward and dorsal pressure on the thyroid cartilage. A less-invasive approach is to begin the process of experiencing the new lower pitch through the device of utilising vegetative vocal function, a cough or a laugh or a grunt, and explaining the relevance of this note to the patient. It should be stated that voice therapy is an effective treatment for MF patients with laryngeal hyperfunction. Most MF patients can return to normal voice in 4 weeks. Vocal aerodynamic examination can help in predicting the voice therapy effect and deciding the treatment plan (Liang *et al.*, 2017). MF patients without laryngeal hyperfunction may need a longer voice therapy period or other adjuvant treatment (Varma *et al.*, 2015). Whichever approach is used it is then possible to work with the patient to encourage an extension of the note through prolongation into a vowel or indeed a hum and from there into single phonemes, simple words, phrases and short sentences. An alternative surgical approach (Pau and Murty, 2001) achieves the result of lowering the larynx with a concomitant lowering of the pitch. Vaidya and Vyas (2006) report on a successful study which caused an immediate change from child to adult voice through the application of pressure to the valleculae with a laryngoscope and digital manipulation of the thyroid cartilage.

Once the patient has achieved a lower note it is important to reinforce the 'new' voice and validate the sound as acceptable to the patient. Treatment should ensure that the new voice is stabilised as quickly as possible, but generalisation of the 'new' voice may need to be a gradual process. It is important to prepare the patient for comments and questions as these may well occur, and to encourage the patient to try to ignore any negative comments by others on the 'new' voice. The idea is to facilitate the route to acceptance for the patient if necessary, but of course some patients report very positively on the changed attitude of friends or that 'no one noticed'. Strategies to consolidate the use of the new voice may include the completion of a number of clinician-directed assignments. These will depend on the patient's personal, cultural and ethnic environment and should be decided in conjunction with the patient.

Organic voice disorders

Structural

Into this category fall voice disorders that are caused by physical changes in the vocal mechanism from vocal fold tissue change, trauma to the larynx or inflammation of the larynx, such as laryngitis, nodules, polyps, cysts, oedema, contact ulcers, granuloma, dysplasia, papilloma, laryngeal web, haemorrhage, sulcus vocalis, traumatic injury or scarring. Chapter 3 will focus on these conditions individually, describing the nature of the lesion and the effect on vocal fold vibration and on voice quality. Because many of the laryngeal conditions above may be secondary to a Muscle Tension Dysphonia (MTD), this section should be considered along with MTD.

The primary cause of vocal misuse and in effect the primary characteristic of trauma to the larynx is the hyper adduction of the extrinsic and intrinsic laryngeal musculature frequently accompanied by excessive vocal fold tension. Deem and Miller (2000) suggest the term 'behavioural', or 'phonotrauma', for this type of dysphonia. As a result of this excessive laryngeal tension, changes in laryngeal tissue may occur – namely alterations to the mass, elasticity and tension of the vocal folds. Oedema and haematoma of the vocal folds (submucosal swelling caused by a collection of fluid or blood, respectively) due to laryngeal trauma, such as intubation, may resolve spontaneously, but repeated episodes will have the secondary effect of a build-up of granular deposits on the vocal folds, with eventual fibrosis leading to polyps and nodules. The resulting vocal quality is generally hoarse, husky, breathy or low-pitched. Whatever term is used, trauma to the laryngeal tissue which results in voice quality change can be the result of one isolated episode of vocal misuse but, more usually, is the result of extended periods of vocal misuse.

Direct trauma to the larynx can occur when the patient receives a blow to the laryngeal area as a result of road traffic accidents, assault or sport injuries. This may cause oedema, structural damage, or both, with subsequent change in voice quality. It is imperative for the patient to receive advice during the immediate post-traumatic period so that no further MTD evolves to complicate and prolong recovery.

Neurological

In this category fall voice disorders that are caused by a neurological disorder such as paralysis/paresis, spasmodic dysphonia, tremor and voice problems caused by another neurological disorder such as Parkinson's disease or myasthenia gravis. Chapter 3 will give a description of various voice disorders of a neurological aetiology and the impact on voice production and quality of the voice.

Given the nature and aetiology of neurological voice disorders, it is most important that an accurate diagnosis is made as soon as possible so that the clinician, patient, General Practitioner, family members and significant others can be informed regarding the likely prognosis and potential treatment options. In some instances, diagnosis may be immediate during an Ear, Nose and Throat examination, as in vocal fold paralysis/paresis where the changes in the laryngeal structure and function can be clearly observed. The confirmation of aetiology may take longer. However in, for example, spasmodic dysphonia or progressive disorders, diagnosis cannot always be immediate, as the patient requires specialist consultations and examinations to determine the precise aetiology of the disorder.

Because a change in voice quality may often be an early or one of the first symptoms of some of the above progressive neurological disorders (Carding, 2003; Sidor, 2010), the voice clinician may receive referral information, which describes various symptoms from MTD to roughness or weakness of voice. The case history and full assessment of the patient is therefore an integral part of the patient journey towards accurate diagnosis. The voice clinician may be the first person to notice tremor, change in facial expression, disordered resonance, symptoms of dysarthria or dysphagia, or change in balance or gait. It is then important that the locally approved route is followed for ongoing referral, whether that is through the General Practitioner, ENT consultant or directly to the Neurologist.

Clearly the whole process towards diagnosis is highly sensitive and should be handled carefully by, or with the guidance of, an experienced clinician, because the ultimate diagnosis and prognosis will determine the best treatment options and management of the patient. When diagnosis has been confirmed, this can be discussed with the patient, those closest to him/her and with representatives of support groups if appropriate.

Other groups for consideration

Professional/occupational voice users

This group of voice users may also be classified in the Structural or Functional categories, dependent on the laryngeal condition.

The term 'professional voice user' carries with it an implicit expectation that individuals will have had training to bring their vocal skills up to a 'professional' level and, by training, expertise and ability, their vocal skills allow them to use their voice effectively in a variety of settings and to different numbers and groups of people (Martin and Darnley, 2019). Increasingly this group of 'professional voice users' present with what is now more commonly termed 'occupational voice disorders' and it is this overarching term that the author has chosen to use in this publication. 'Occupational voice user' is used here to refer to those individuals whose professional role and employment are dependent on effective and efficient use of voice. In this group, for example, may be included teachers, actors, politicians, call centre workers, radio announcers, clergy, barristers, dealers on the stock exchange, priests, auctioneers and sales people.

Fortunately, some health authorities recognise the need to 'fast track' professional or occupational voice users to a speech and language therapy-led Endoscopy Clinic. Usually the criterion for referral and assessment at such clinics is agreed by the local Ear, Nose and Throat

Directorate, with a potential route to secondary advice and further examination built into the patient journey. Similarly, it is usual for a stringent monitoring process to be in place; for example, the laryngeal endoscopy may be digitally recorded and documented so that it can be reviewed by the ENT consultant or an experienced SLT. This maintains high-quality service provision, is cost-effective, contributes to clinical efficacy and efficiency, supports the professional supervision process and is a robust means of ensuring and demonstrating continuing competence by the clinician fulfilling the endoscopy. This will be discussed further in Chapter 8.

Concern has existed for many years that those who fall into the 'occupational voice user' category are ill-served by either training or legislation to support their vocal needs. Gilman *et al.* (2009) raise the important issue of lack of awareness among professional singers about the specialised voice care services available from laryngologists and SLTs. While most of the participants in their study indicated that their voice was very important to their profession, they were less likely to seek help for vocal problems than for general health problems. While their study was conducted in the USA, its findings are not USA-centric, as it is not only singers who are unaware of the services which are available but also occupational voice users. Many occupational voice users such as teachers increasingly form a disproportionately large number of patients attending voice therapy. Studies from the USA and Europe demonstrate that no particular teacher group is immune from the voice problems which relate to its professional role. In the USA, information from the University of Iowa (2017) stated that, working on the evidence of a study by Dr Katherine Verdolini and Dr Lorraine Ramig, the cost of teachers' voice problems on an annual basis was $2.5 billion. This figure included medical costs, pharmacy and insurance expenses, plus the cost of employing supply teachers. Teachers are about 4% of the US workforce yet constitute almost 20% of the patient load in voice clinics. Given that at that time there were 5,168,000 US teachers of which approximately 40% experience voice problems, that would seem to indicate that 2,067,200 teachers have hoarseness, vocal fatigue or other voice difficulties, yet of the group only 15% actually sought treatment. Similarly, in the United Kingdom, many fewer teachers who experience voice loss report a problem or seek treatment. Anecdotal evidence suggests that they feel that doing so might label them as professionally vulnerable. Studies confirm a consistently high world-wide incidence of voice problems within the teaching population in comparison to other occupations (Morton and Watson, 1998; De Jong *et al.*, 2006; Preciado-Lopez *et al.*, 2008; Martin and Darnley, 2019). These studies span over 20 years, several different countries and two continents, yet the figure remains remarkably consistent and mirrors findings from studies of vocal attrition going back for almost five decades; for examples, see Cooper (1973) and Herrington-Hall *et al.* (1988).

The very nature of occupational voice use presents specific challenges in terms of remedi-ation, because while voice therapy is usually successful and treatment options are predicated on evidence-based therapy, the continual high level of vocal loading experienced by the occupational voice user as part of their professional roles can jeopardise recovery. Clearly reduction in vocal loading is essential, but in the author's opinion, total voice rest for these patients is not the optimal choice. Mathieson (2001) suggests that complete voice rest is only imperative in the case of vocal fold haemorrhage and is not convinced that absolute voice rest offers better protection post-operatively than a programme of voice conserva-tion. Behrman and Sulica (2003) studied voice rest and their results indicated a preference for the use of voice rest for an average of seven days regardless of the type of lesion. Voice rest can place heavy and sometimes unrealistic demands on the patient. It is certainly dif-ficult to supervise and 'police' and does little to change vocal behaviours that contributed to the vocal condition in the first place. Some patients may indeed refuse to agree to voice rest (Behlau *et al.*, 2009). A study by Whitling *et al.* (2018) looked at the benefit of absolute voice rest (AVR) following phonosurgery and compared the benefit of absolute voice rest to relative voice rest (RVR) and concluded that 'AVR may be fruitful for short term histological recovery but long term benefits were not shown in this study'. They go on to conclude that 'patients recommended for RVR showed significantly better vocal stamina and immediate recovery from vocal loading' at long-term follow-up.

Clinicians must make their own decisions about the value of AVR and take into consideration the unintended consequence of potentially 'pathologising' the patient. It may well be more realistic to advise patients to reduce the amount of talking that they do, and encourage vocal conservation in terms of soft onset, reduced loudness and avoidance of abusive vocal behaviours such as throat clearing.

Gender dysphoria

Almost four decades ago, Oates and Dacakis (1983) published the first general framework for voice therapy with patients with Gender Dysphoria (GD) in which they recommended that not only should voice therapy be directed to changing fundamental frequency characteristics but also in achieving maximum effectiveness. They suggested that voice therapy should also be directed towards vocal features such as prosody, intensity, voice quality and resonance. While there is now much more knowledge of and information on the needs of trans men, trans women and non-binary individuals, Oates in 2012 commented on the lack of data-based research papers and regretted the continued lack of evidence of outcome measures. Oates' view was that many of these were, in general, weak in terms of the research hierarchy; a view reinforced by the work of Davies *et al.* (2015) in their review of current research. Investigation of the best existing measures (including examination of pre- and post-treatment change, with more rigorous peer-reviewed research to inform clinical research and practice) remains limited. Stoneham and Mills (2017) suggest that a brief but broad repeatable measure for progress monitoring, which would cover key aspects of gender congruence, experience of and coping around stigma and discrimination, community connection and social support, plus general well-being, would foster substantive improvements in treatment and research with transgender gender non-conforming (TGNC) individuals.

The question of whether it is essential to have a robust evidence base as a precursor to treatment is an interesting one, as to some extent this reflects much of the work of the voice clinician where limited evidence-based studies are available, despite the best efforts of researchers, an issue raised almost 20 years ago by Carding (2003).

Stoneham and Mills (2017) affirm that 'voice and communication therapy, also known as voice modification therapy, is delivered by speech and language therapists in order to assist trans and gender-diverse people in creating and sustaining their authentic voice and communication, congruent with their sense of self'. Many clinicians will never work with trans clients, although in the face of growing identification and need this is changing and clinicians need to be prepared to seek advice and support from clinically skilled and experienced therapists as access for patients to specialist gender identity clinics (GIC) may well outstrip provision. The multidisciplinary team approach offered in a GIC is, in the author's view, strongly recommended, as the complexity of the issues which need to be considered (medical, surgical, psychological and socio-cultural) require a collaborative approach. This allows intervention by, for example, surgeon, psychiatrist, social worker, endocrinologist, specialist nurse, counsellor and clinician, thus ensuring intervention is seamless and effective with joint sharing of information and expertise. In the UK the Royal College of Speech and Language Therapists established a National Transgender Voice and Communication Therapy Clinical Excellence Network (CEN) in 2016 and a competency framework for Speech and Language Therapists is in process, which will support clinicians working on their own. It is, however, important to consider how critical gender congruence really is – the objective surely is for voice to be part of the individual, not an 'over lay' to a gender change.

The conceptualisation and assessment of the psychological experience of identifying as TGNC has advanced considerably over the last 40 years (Shulman *et al.*, 2017). Despite the plethora of research documenting that the voice and quality of life (QoL) are related, the exact nature of this relationship is vague. Studies have not addressed people who consider their voice to influence their life and identity but would not be considered to have a voice 'disorder' (e.g. transgender individuals). Individuals seeking vocal feminisation may or may not have vocal pathology and often have concerns not addressed on the standard psycho-social measures of voice impact. The development of a voice-related QoL measure specific to the needs of transgender care, the Transgender Self-Evaluation Questionnaire (Hancock *et al.*, 2010) affords an opportunity to explore relationships between self-perceived QoL and perceptions of femininity and likability, associated with transgender voice. For male-to-female transgender clients, QoL is moderately correlated with how others perceive their voice. QoL ratings correlate more strongly with a speaker's self-rated perception of voice compared with others' perceptions, more so for likability than femininity.

Voice modification therapy should focus on patient-specific goals for transgender clients. The goals most often recommended in the research literature focus on voice and communication treatment. These elements are usually those deemed most highly salient to gender attribution, which include: fundamental frequency, resonance, intonation, volume and intensity, breath support, speaking rate, language, pragmatics and vocal health. In addition to providing voice therapy, clinicians working with transgender individuals also often work on the non-verbal aspects of communication, such as eye contact and facial expression.

A warning caveat comes from Colton *et al.* (2011), who suggest that the goal of therapy is 'to make those changes that will be effective in changing the overall image, rather than to work on artificial changes such as pitch change, that may never become natural and that in fact may court laryngeal problems'. This, as has already been noted, should be seen through the prism of gender congruence rather than a fixed goal of achieving gender/voice synchronicity.

There is the potential for transgender clients to cause damage to their vocal folds if they try to push out sounds that their voices can't make, so the work of the clinician in this field also includes identifying any underlying vocal pathologies, educating clients on proper vocal care, and overseeing the process of making gradual and subtle voice changes over time.

It is encouraging to know that voice and communication treatment for patients with gender dysphoria is generally effective, but measures of how communication partners perceive the speaker's gender would be most useful in order to determine the effectiveness of the ultimate goal, namely, passing as the desired gender. As noted above, further research is warranted to determine the efficacy of specific treatment protocols and potentially influential factors such as initial voice and communication status.

The Transsexual Voice Questionnaire for Male-to-Female Transsexuals (TVQ MtF; Dacakis *et al.*, 2013) is a self-report tool designed to capture an individual's perception of her voice and how it impacts on her everyday life. It is a population-specific tool for individuals whose female gender identity is the opposite to that of their birth-assigned gender.

Fewer transgender males seek voice and communication therapy than transgender females, generally because the desired change in pitch is often achieved through hormone therapy. Gender judgements based on voice for female-to-male (FtM) TGNC patients has received less attention than that of MtF patients, which could mean that for these individuals fundamental frequency is a relatively less important factor for gender expression than is the case with MtF TGNC individuals (Van Borsel *et al.*, 2009). Andrews (2006) suggests that 'females moving along the path to male gender identity rarely consult speech pathologists'. If voice and communication therapy is required it is undertaken alongside medical/surgical interventions and hormone therapy, but often vocal change is managed satisfactorily solely through the use of hormone administration. It must, of course, be remembered that hormone therapy is essential for all TGNC patients and clinicians are directed to visit specific websites for up-to-date information on hormone therapy because drug regimens and treatment options are frequently reviewed and refined. In the case of all MtF patients feminising hormone therapy is given while FtM patients will follow a masculinising hormone regimen resulting in an increase in laryngeal mass and size and a consequent lowering of fundamental frequency. While appropriate pitch is important in the perception of gender, it is, in fact, worth noting that there is considerable overlap in the pitch range of men and women and work on fundamental frequency as such should not always be the ultimate goal. As clinicians will be aware, there are other feminine speech markers that in addition to the pitch differences are equally, if not more, important. These include pitch variability and increased vocal variety. Work on pitch variability, stereotypical feminine intonation patterns such as rising inflections at the ends of some utterances and resonance would seem to offer a more all-encompassing approach. Dacakis (2000), Freidenberg (2002) and Oates (2012) target work on encouraging 'oral' and 'head' resonance, minimising 'chest' resonance, feminising coughing, throat clearing and laughing, imitation of female voice models, self-monitoring, generalising of voice skills through a hierarchy of role-play and transfer tasks as areas for change.

While voice training procedures are one route for the MtF TGNC patient, surgical intervention is another. Laryngeal surgery may be effective to help to raise vocal pitch, but as with any surgery the procedure is not without risk. A three-year follow-up study of a Type IV thyroplasty (Gibbons *et al.*, 2011) reported findings of increased pitch definition and clarity but decreased range overall. Surgery, however, will not always be available to patients, and clinicians may have MtF transition patients referred who have not had, and will not have, surgery.

It should always be remembered when working with the TGNC patient that the clinician needs to be aware of their role within the transition process while, as Mordaunt (2012) says, 'constantly adhering to ethical and professional regulations. The balance between professionalism and compassion can sometimes be difficult'. Dacakis (2006) suggests that the clinician should be aware that the management of the TGNC patient involves 'as many similarities to the management of "everyday" disorders as it involves stark differences'.

Clinicians need to consider the whole person, bringing a unique level of understanding of both the psychological and physiological implications of gender transition. Therapy provision may be offered at any point during transition, or even in the years following.

Capturing the individual's self-perception of their voice and its impact on everyday life is acknowledged as an important component of voice assessment (Dacakis *et al.*, 2013; Stemple *et al.*, 2013). Self-report tools are particularly important when assessing the vocal needs of the MtF woman as clinician evaluations of her voice do not necessarily reflect how her voice impacts on her everyday life (Remacle *et al.*, 2011).

Exercises to address aspects of vocal care and safe vocal change are to be found in Chapter 7 under the headings of posture, relaxation, breathing, voice, pitch, resonance and muscular flexibility, and will address:

- muscle tension in the head, neck and larynx;
- breath control and support to target increasing breath support and control while speaking;
- vocal hygiene to include advice on hydration, amount and intensity of daily voice use and, occasionally, reflux precautions;
- reduction of specific phonotraumatic behaviour, like hard attack;
- easy onset of voice.

Inducible laryngeal obstruction

Inducible Laryngeal Dysfunction (ILO), or Vocal Cord Dysfunction (VCD), typically involves abnormal adduction of the vocal folds during inspiration and mimics the symptoms of asthma with intermittent wheeze and dyspnoea. It often follows exposure to triggers such as exercise, chemicals and odours, causing laryngeal irritation, rhinitis or sinusitis (Morris and Christopher, 2010). The pathophysiology of VCD is poorly understood and it is sometimes considered to be more a psychological disorder. Certainly psychological factors sometimes play a role in the presentation of ILO, but there is now greater recognition of other contributing factors such as LPR, GORD and underlying lung and nasal disease which may be a trigger for ILO. The Vocal Cord Dysfunction Questionnaire (VCDQ; Fowler *et al.*, 2015) is a questionnaire for symptom monitoring in vocal cord dysfunction and was developed to monitor response to speech and language therapy and further treatment developments.

Traister *et al.* (2016) looked at the morbidity and cost of VCD misdiagnosed as asthma and determined that misdiagnosis of VCD as asthma leads to significant morbidity and increased costs, and misuse of measures of asthma control may be contributing to these findings. They suggest that timely and accurate diagnosis of VCD and the use of breathing exercises have the potential to eliminate or minimise symptoms for the patient. They identified symptoms of shortness of breath, wheezing, chest tightness and a trigger of exercise as being more common in the subjects with VCD misdiagnosed as asthma. They recommend breathing exercises as an effective and inexpensive treatment for patients with VCD. Fajt *et al.* (2018) noted the co-existence of VCD with pulmonary conditions other than asthma and highlighted the fact that VCD cannot only mimic or co-exist with asthma but can also co-exist with other pulmonary conditions. The patient's failure to respond to common treatment modalities should alert the clinician to search for alternative diagnoses.

Halvorsen (2017) noted the following as the most commonly recognised symptoms in ILO:

- wheezing/coughing;
- a feeling of tightness in the throat;
- hoarseness and voice change;
- stridor;
- shortness of breath;
- dyspnoea;
- inspiratory difficulty;
- sudden episodes of shortness of breath;
- unresponsiveness to bronchodilators and corticosteroids.

Psychological mechanisms may have wide implications for various presentations of ILO. Generally, treatment strategies are aimed at avoidance of exposure to presumed inducers or represent methods for improved coping, including psychotherapy or psychological counselling. Psychotherapy or psychological counselling is often accompanied by voice therapy and described with biofeedback. According to Fowler *et al.* (2015), there existed a level of ignorance of the condition among speech and language therapists but this is no longer the case, with intervention now aimed at treatments such as nasal breathing, panting and diaphragmatic breathing, focusing attention away from the larynx and refocusing attention to a specific task (e.g. exercise). Haines *et al.* (2018) report that 'despite recent advances, knowledge and understanding of ILO remains limited'. The researchers go on to suggest that there are some important deficiencies in current knowledge in the field, concluding that it is essential that these are addressed systematically in future research to facilitate improved care for patients.

Chronic cough

Chronic cough is defined as a cough that persists despite guideline-based treatment (Gibson and Vertigan, 2015). The Royal College of Speech and Language Therapists website (www.rcslt.org) affirms that 'All people with idiopathic or refractory chronic cough and ILO should have access to an appropriate respiratory Speech and Language Therapy service' (accessed 29 March 2020).

The symptoms most commonly recognised in chronic cough are:

- dry irritated cough;
- globus;
- dyspnoea;
- dysphonia.

The pathophysiology of chronic cough includes cough reflex sensitivity, central sensitisation, peripheral sensitisation and VCD with, it is suggested, 8–10% of the adult population experiencing chronic cough (Song *et al.*, 2015). This is not to be confused with a persistent dry cough that can be the side effect of prescription drugs from the ACE inhibitor family, used to mitigate high blood pressure, for example, Ramipril or perindopril.

It is the experience of the author that it is not unusual for patients to be referred with dysphonia precipitated by chronic cough, which becomes a precipitating and perpetuating factor in the dysphonia. Few effective medical treatments are known, but suggested intervention is a combination of voice therapy, with an emphasis on vocal hygiene to teach techniques to reduce the trigger to cough, plus neuromodulators such as a bronchodilator like ipratropium bromide which demonstrates a reduction in cough severity and a good safety profile. The combination acts on different aspects of the cough pathway, thus providing a more complete response. While this approach improves the cough it does not eliminate it, as neuromodulators are limited by side effects and non-sustained treatment response. Vertigan *et al.* (2006) showed speech and language therapy is an effective management and intervention for chronic cough that may be a viable alternative for patients who do not respond to medical treatment, but in a recent Cochrane review a lack of high-quality, relevant studies has limited their ability to support SLT intervention unequivocally (Slinger *et al.*, 2019). Chronic cough is recognised as having a severe impact on a patient's quality of life; the Leicester Cough Questionnaire (LCQ; Birring *et al.*, 2003) is one of a number of self-completed, health-related, quality-of-life measures of chronic cough and may be used in the clinical assessment of treatment efficacy. Some suggestions for therapy for both VCD and chronic cough are included in Chapter 7.

Aerophagia

Aerophagia has been described as the initial presenting symptom of anxiety and depression in a patient (Appleby and Rosenburg, 2006). It is usually defined as a condition where a person swallows too much air, too frequently, in too large quantities which results in constant and/or excessive belching or burping. The swallowed air goes into the stomach and/or oesophagus and may or may not be associated with digestive upset. It is often thought to be associated with food allergies and GORD. Modification of eating patterns and respiratory intervention has been very successful when working with patients. However, a study of 79 patients with aerophagia and 121 patients with upper gastrointestinal symptoms reports distinctly different symptoms in the two groups (Chitkara *et al.*, 2005), with the patients with aerophagia having an average duration of the disorder of 24 months.

Lockhart (2009) reported that some patients with aerophagia appear to be following an air-intake process very similar to that of the laryngectomee/oesophageal voice user. Air may be compressed into the oesophagus through a 'pumping' movement of the tongue and expelled as a burp. This may be associated with stress, muscular hypertension and a tendency to press the tongue against the hard palate. In some patients, the frequency of burping may be almost constant and exceedingly distressing and embarrassing to the patient and his/her family. In those patients where stress, anxiety and muscular tension appear to be associated with the aerophagia, treatment by the voice clinician can be very successful. Lockhart (2009) reported significant success in alleviating the disorder through therapy targeting relaxation of the oral, pharyngeal, laryngeal and respiratory muscle function. Modification of eating, breathing patterns and attention to underlying conditions such as anxiety has been found to be effective and is to be recommended, although it is not a condition, however, that is often treated in voice clinics.

Summary

Classification of voice disorders is an evolving issue. There may eventually be one universal system to which all clinicians will subscribe, but at the time of writing this is still not the case, so following personal choice the DCSVD classification was used in this chapter and the next.

What is not in question, however, is the increasing acknowledgement of the impact of psychosocial factors in the aetiology of many forms of functional dysphonia due to an association with anxiety, grief and depression. While Aronson and Moses established this connection over 60 years ago and others have followed over the decades, there has been an encouraging increase in and recognition of this connection from the wider ENT community, highlighted in this chapter. The work of the clinician in preventative work with occupational voice users has been equally encouraging, as has the expanding role of the clinician in the diagnosis and treatment of ILO and chronic cough. The challenge of this chapter was to inform and orientate readers to the spectrum of voice disorders and to certain discrete and unique groups. Other voice disorders exist, but it is to be hoped that those most commonly encountered on clinical caseloads have all been included.

3

THE SPECTRUM OF VOICE DISORDERS - PRESENTATION

Introduction

Where Chapter 2 explored the spectrum of voice disorders and its classification, this chapter will outline the vocal fold movement patterns or organic changes corresponding to the Voice Disorder classification. Where there is an organic disorder, the impairment to voice involves a lesion of the phonatory system, which may be congenital, inflammatory, traumatic, neoplastic or neurological.

In the following pages are practical descriptions of common types of disorders found in most clinicians' caseloads and summarised in Table 3.1 at the end of this chapter. Detail is provided of the vocal symptoms, the appearance of the vocal folds at the free fold edge, the expected vibration patterns in the mucosal wave, a description of the typical dysphonia produced and the options for therapy.

Functional voice disorders – muscle tension dysphonia

Posterior glottic chink (PGC)

When the posterior cricoarytenoid muscles are consistently contracted with increased tension, the posterior part of the vocal folds sit in an open position, allowing air to escape during phonation, resulting in a breathy voice with the potential for further increased muscle tension within the larynx. Hypertonicity within the larynx and stiffness of the vocal folds may lead to reduced mucosal wave on videostroboscopy. PGC may occur in those who report no voice disorder but who have a relatively 'gentle' and somewhat breathy voice. It is important that a distinction is made between what is 'normal' and what is a 'pathology' by the clinician, as in fact incomplete closure of the posterior part of the vocal folds is a common factor in young and middle-aged women (Sodersten *et al.*, 1995). PGC is, however, often associated with occupational voice users, those who use voice professionally or occupationally and who have poor voice production technique and/or high level of voice demand. Treatment should focus on precipitating and perpetuating factors and improved voice technique.

Morrison and Rammage (2000) describe PGC as the 'laryngeal isometric', which is frequently associated with palpable increase in suprahyoid muscle tension on phonation, particularly in higher pitch ranges. They suggest that 'strong adduction forces employed to overcome exaggerated abduction in the posterior glottis lead to greater shearing stress on the mid-membranous vocal folds at the position where nodules typically develop'.

Lateral constriction and/or hyperadduction

Lateral laryngeal constriction has been described as 'a type of tension fatigue syndrome in which the larynx tends to be squeezed or hyperadducted in a side to side direction. It may exist either at the glottic or supraglottic level' (Morrison and Rammage, 2000). The precipitating factors vary from upper respiratory tract infections (URTI) to anxiety and psychogenic influences. The vocal folds, and sometimes also the supraglottic muscles, contract in this 'squeezing' manner during phonation, producing a tense and forced vocal quality. The mucosal wave pattern during vibration may be reduced due to muscle stiffness. Although, as mentioned, this may be related to anxiety or the discomfort and coughing/throat-clearing symptoms of URTI, it can also be associated with a high level of voice demand in occupational voice users and the need to use voice for lengthy periods of time with few rest periods (Titze *et al.*, 2007; Hunter and Titze, 2009). Not surprisingly, patients report discomfort in the neck and larynx as well as vocal fatigue and disturbance to breathing patterns. Attention to the disordered vocal technique and voice management is necessary. Vocal loading advice is essential.

Anteroposterior contraction of the supraglottic larynx

Kooijman *et al.* (2005) suggest that laryngeal elevation may increase anterior-posterior (AP) supraglottic contraction which in turn can affect vocal fold vibratory patterns. Patients present with a low-pitched voice, report fatigue and increased effort to produce voice, but are able to talk more clearly and more freely at a higher pitch. Singers may exhibit a similar AP contraction pattern on phonation in association with tense pharyngolaryngeal postures. Treatment focus should be on reducing the general tension in the neck and larynx, lowering the habitual laryngeal position and facilitating improved voice techniques with appropriate pitch placement.

Ventricular phonation

Despite its low incidence, ventricular phonation is a well-known phenomenon in voice clinics. Maryn and Bodt (2003) refer to it as 'pathological interference of the false folds during phonation'. The term may be used to mean complete adduction of the ventricular folds during phonation or partial (hyperadduction) during phonation. In both there may be hypertrophy and/or hyperadduction of the ventricular (false) folds resulting in low-pitched, forced and rough voice with the possibility of diplophonia and fatigue, as true voice and ventricular voice are produced in synchrony. The ventricular folds appear hyperadducted, bulky and inflamed, often concealing the true vocal folds. Maryn *et al.* (2009) suggest that there may be various aetiologies of this disorder, including compensatory factors when, for example, the true vocal folds are affected by resection or paralysis, or from non-compensatory features such as habitual psycho-emotional or idiopathic origin; indeed, any condition which reduces the adequacy of voice for the required phonatory environment. The prognosis for improvement of voice quality is closely linked with the aetiology of the disorder and a careful case history is most important in determining not only the causative factors, but also the treatment strategies for achieving the reduction in excessive vocal effort. Intervention should reduce the hyperadduction of the ventricular folds by the appropriate therapeutic techniques. Colton *et al.* (2011) suggest that when ventricular phonation is associated with a psychogenic origin it can be easily reversed, but when the true vocal folds are incapable of adduction, ventricular phonation appears to be a compensatory mechanism that is very resistant to change.

Bowing of the vocal folds (vocal fold atrophy)

Loss of tension in the vocal fold muscles results in the 'bowed' shape along the free edge and in poor approximation of the fold edges during vibration. Voice may become breathy and weak and may be higher in pitch where there is thinning of the vocal folds. This can be caused by various aetiologies, such as vocal fold paralysis and sulcus vocalis; chronic misuse and overloading of the voice can also result in muscle fatigue, loss of muscle elasticity and thinning of the vocal folds. It is a common presenting symptom in those who have used excessive vocal energy over many years, or who have sung regularly at a pitch which is too high. The vocal fold muscles become fatigued with loss of elasticity and are unable to fulfil normal closure and function during vibration. They appear to 'flap' rather than to vibrate and have poor mucosal wave. Although this condition may not resolve completely with therapy, it is possible to reduce the muscle energy expended and facilitate the best voice possible, while limiting further damage. LaGoria *et al.* (2010) reported that behavioural voice therapy with adjunctive neuromuscular electrical stimulation reduced vocal fold bowing and resulted in improved acoustic, laryngeal and glottal closure results.

Bowing – ageing voice

With older age come generalised changes in respiration and phonation due to postural change, reduction in respiratory competence and strength, changes in the vocal fold muscles, loss of tension and resonance changes, as well as the impact of reduced levels of hyaluronic acid on vocal fold function. These are described in Chapter 1. However, this is not inevitable and many individuals continue to have strong and resonant voice in older age. Where changes in voice do occur due to natural or premature ageing, there is often reduction in vocal agility and changes in vocal quality such as reduced resonance, pitch breaks and lack of vocal intensity with inadequate breath support for normal sentence length. Similarly, articulatory imprecision may contribute to the listener's perception of a disorder.

On examination, the vocal folds show loss of tension and possibly some pigmentation changes with little mucosal wave. The clinician should advise on reduction of misuse while ensuring optimal voice adequacy.

Bowing of the vocal folds due to neurological disorder will be discussed later in this chapter.

Psychogenic voice disorders/conversion aphonia

Hyperadduction/hyperabduction

Due to the nature of psychogenic voice disorder, there are many and varied presenting symptoms including those described in the section on MTD. When the vocal folds and/or supraglottic area exhibit hypertonicity and hyperadduction, the voice is squeezed, effortful and easily fatigued. It may also be high-pitched and 'squeaky'. There may be little audible airflow or, in some patients, no airflow or ingressive airflow. Some patients may produce normal phonation occasionally for a syllable or two within a phrase as the muscles relax intermittently. Normal phonation is also often heard on spontaneous, interjected words or vegetative sounds. This type of aphonia may also be a form of 'habitual hoarseness' (Morrison and Rammage, 2000) which follows an URTI or other organic trigger. When the vocal folds are hyperabducted, there is an absence of phonation. Communication may be whispered with outgoing airflow or may be with no airflow as the patient attempts to speak while 'holding the breath'.

As noted earlier, standard voice therapy alone for the management of Psychogenic Voice Disorders and Functional Voice Disorders has begun to lose favour (Butcher *et al.*, 2007). As a consequence, a combination of voice therapy with psychological therapies is recommended. Clearly, the decision depends on the careful assessment of the aetiology, precipitating and perpetuating factors. Therapy for this patient group is discussed in Chapter 2.

Organic voice disorders - structural

Laryngitis

Acute laryngitis should be of short duration and associated with upper respiratory tract infection, influenza or viral infection. The vocal folds may be inflamed and oedematous, resulting in moderate to severe dysphonia/aphonia caused by the upper respiratory tract infection. Shah (2016) suggests that this dysphonia/aphonia is usually self-limiting; recovery will occur with appropriate treatment of the underlying condition with no need for referral for voice treatment.

Chronic laryngitis is a more persistent disorder and is rarely caused by an inflammatory illness or an infection such as sarcoidosis or tuberculosis related to the vocal folds. As noted by Khidr *et al.* (2003), the laryngeal symptoms are most commonly caused by vocal misuse, for example, laryngeal irritation from exposure to chemicals, dust, smoking, alcohol abuse, GORD or LPR (Allen *et al.*, 2019). In addition, irritation due to hypersensitivity type of occupational laryngitis (OL) has been noted by Hannu *et al.* (2009). Less often, chronic laryngitis is caused by chronic sinusitis with post-nasal drip.

In the case of chronic laryngitis the vocal folds may appear thickened, slightly oedematous or with some irregularity of the free vocal fold edge and will present with stiffness which results in reduced amplitude of vibration and lack of mucosal wave. The patient's voice may be lowered in pitch, breathy and/or rough with a pattern of hyperfunctional voice having evolved during the course of the disorder, as increased effort is associated with voice use. With therapeutic intervention and patient compliance, the vocal fold condition should resolve and voice should return to normal quality and function. Where this does not take place and the condition continues, there is the possibility of the continuing laryngeal irritation leading to vocal nodules and/or chronic oedema of the vocal folds.

Vocal nodules

Impact stress on the vocal folds during phonation and the effect of maximal impact in the mid-membranous vocal fold may lead to pathological changes within the superficial layer of the lamina propria. As a consequence, at the point of greatest impact on the vocal fold edge (the anterior third and posterior two-thirds), unilateral or bilateral nodules may form.

Vocal nodules are the result of vocal misuse, often due to excessive vocal loading with too short a recovery phase and inadequacy of the vocal system to sustain such demand. It can also be the result of the habitual use of inappropriate pitch placement or too high a volume of voice without adequate voice production/support. Constant coughing, acid reflux or allergies can also cause similar phonotrauma leading to chronic localised trauma to the vocal mucosa, which is often compared to chronic wound healing (Hunter and Titze, 2009). Vocal fold masses including polyps, nodules, Reinke's space and cysts are usually benign, but this is not always the case as it will depend on the histological degeneration present (Altman, 2007).

Vocal nodules often result in a breathy and effortful voice with breaks in phonation and in pitch. There may be a deterioration of voice during the day as the vocal folds become progressively more irritated or oedematous and vocal effort is increased, precipitating a MTD. Throat clearing is a common symptom as the patient reports a feeling of 'something in my throat'.

Nodules may be small and/or soft, producing little disturbance to the vocal fold vibration and may reduce well with vocal rehabilitation. Depending on the type and size of the nodule, there may be disturbance to the vibratory patterns of the vocal folds and the mucosal wave. However, on videostroboscopy, antero-posterior compression/contraction and stiffness of the vocal folds is often noted.

With regular voice therapy, vocal hygiene advice such as the reduction of irritants, alteration of vocal behaviours and rehabilitation of the muscle tension disorder, the prognosis for recovery of voice should be good and the possibility of recurrence reduced. Phonomicrosurgery may be a treatment option.

Vocal fold polyps

Vocal fold polyps are benign growths of the vocal fold which are usually unilateral. They are the result of vocal misuse and phonotrauma, in many cases with excessive smoking, alcohol or GORD as contributing influences, but may also be caused by a single or repeated submucous haemorrhages, which leads to polyp formation. Polyps occur on the free edge of the vocal fold and may be small or large, broad-based or peduncular.

Polyps may require a combination of surgery and voice intervention depending on the site and type of polyp. Similarly, the disturbance to vocal fold vibration may be considerable or insignificant. Characteristically the voice is rough and breathy, with pitch and voice breaks as in vocal nodules, sometimes also with diplophonia.

As with vocal nodules, the prognosis for voice recovery is dependent not only on surgery, but also on reducing irritants, eliminating vocal misuse, reducing phonotrauma, looking at improved vocal hygiene and facilitating voice adequacy for all situations. If a polyp is broad-based, the referral diagnosis may be of a vocal nodule. Also, the term 'polypoidal degeneration' may be used to describe Reinke's oedema and should not be confused with the above condition.

Vocal fold cysts

Vocal fold cysts are usually unilateral and may be confused in appearance with vocal nodules or polyps. However, with a vocal fold cyst there is increased stiffness and absence of mucosal wave in the affected vocal fold, which may be detected on videostroboscopy as a valuable aid to diagnosis. Surgery alone is often insufficient as the increased effort to compensate for the lack of vocal closure during vibration may create a secondary muscle tension voice disorder (MTD). Voice therapy can then be very effective in resolving the secondary disorder and enabling normal function and voice recovery.

Some patients may present with no disturbance to voice. However, when there is dysphonia, it may manifest itself as effortful, breathy voice with pitch and phonation breaks. Surgery should be in association with therapy, to reduce any MTD and facilitate optimal voice production. Histology generally shows the cyst lined with columnar or squamous epithelium, and thickened basement membrane zone (BMZ), which is the structurally and biochemically complex junction between the epidermis and dermis.

Reinke's oedema

Reinke's oedema, also known as polypoidal degeneration, involves gelatinous, submucosal oedema of both vocal folds which may not be symmetrical and is often associated with cigarette smoking, LPR and vocal overuse. Reinke's space is fluid-filled, hence the term Reinke's oedema. It is especially common in women over 40 years and is one of the most common benign lesions of the larynx, showing a very low tendency to malignancy.

The laryngeal appearance on videostroboscopy shows no mucosal wave but a gelatinous 'jellyfish' appearance of the vocal folds during vibration. It results in low-pitched, effortful voice, which may also be breathy and rough. Conventional microlaryngoscopic surgery with voice intervention is considered an effective, safe and satisfactory therapy to improve vocal function along with complete cessation of smoking as that induces a recurrence of Reinke's oedema. Salmen *et al.* (2018) recommend that if surgery is undertaken, then a competent and precise microlaryngoscopic excision leaving some gelatinous material in the superficial lamina propria (SLP) is advised along with a normal post-operative course with regular wound healing, vocal rehabilitation, voice intervention and a reduction in vocal irritants.

Unless the underlying causes are treated, Salmen *et al.* (2018) suggest that surgery will be of limited value long-term.

Oedema

Oedema, as an artefact of hypothyroidism, is included here as while in some patients dysphonia may be minimal, in others notable voice changes such as low voice, roughness, reduced rate and vocal fatigue are noted as the surface of the vocal folds may become thickened and asymmetrical with little mucosal wave visible because of the thickening and stiffness of movement during vibration. Changes in the perceptual characteristic of the voice of patients are particularly evident while the acoustic characteristic are less affected by changes. Therefore, Junuzovic-Zunic *et al.* (2019) suggest it is important that changes in the voice of patients with thyroid gland disorders should be carefully assessed and considered. Similarly, vocal fold oedema as a factor in hypothyroidism should be considered even though the vocal parameters are often within normal values. As in many vocal fold disorders, reducing irritants and misuse is required along with therapy to reduce the MTD. There appear to be few follow-up studies on the effect of thyroid hormone replacement therapy on the voices of patients with hypothyroidism.

Contact ulcer

Contact ulcers are erosions of the mucous membrane over the medial surface of the vocal process of the arytenoids cartilages and may be unilateral or bilateral. The vocal folds may be thickened, but generally there is no disturbance to either the mucosal wave or vocal fold vibration. There are various views as to the aetiology of contact ulcers, varying from stress-related factors, gastro-intestinal problems and psychogenic influences to hyperadduction of the vocal folds during phonation and the use of 'creaky' voice or 'vocal fry' as an acquired quality of voice. However, sometimes the patient reports little dysphonia but a sensation of 'something in my throat' with frequent throat clearing or coughing. This may be caused by inflammation or the irritation resulting from GORD or LPR. In some instances a granuloma will form due to the repeated trauma at the site of the lesion during phonation and the impact of hyperadduction on the vocal processes. In long-standing contact ulcers, the granulation of one vocal fold will fit into the depression in the other. Where the case-history data suggest irritants as a precipitating factor, this must be addressed in the patient management. Treatment strategies should also include a reduction in MTD and facilitation of adequate voice production. Voice therapy or proton pump inhibitors (PPIs) are first-line treatments plus Botox. Surgical removal has a significant re-occurrence rate.

Granuloma

(See above for relationship of contact ulcer to granuloma.)

A granuloma, which is a collection of granulated fibrous tissue, may result from trauma to the vocal fold at the vocal process. The lesions typically arise on or near the vocal process of the arytenoids cartilage. They may be caused, for example, from extreme vocal misuse, throat clearing, in association with contact ulcers, due to LPR or intubation during surgery. There may be immediate dysphonia after surgery with discomfort and a persistent cough, at which time advice may be given regarding vocal hygiene and reduced voice use for a short period to allow recovery. An assessment of GORD or LPR and management with pharmacotherapy is advised, as is intervention that focuses on reduction in irritation and on any secondary MTD. Devaney *et al.* (2005) reinforce the view that 'speech therapy is beneficial even if microsurgical therapy with or without CO_2 laser is used'. A granuloma may cause little or no disturbance to voice or to the mucosal wave, but when there is dysphonia it usually results in a breathy, low-pitched, rough voice. More recently Botox Type A injections to treat granulomas have been successful as they temporarily limit the mobility of the vocal fold and reduce vocal misuse, leading to a decrease in irritation and inflammation and allowing the granuloma to heal, as well as preventing new granuloma formation. As the effects of Botox Type A injections are short-lasting (three to five months) they may sometimes be repeated on several occasion to achieve the desired effect. Pham *et al.* (2018) conducted a retrospective chart review and literature review and concluded that in-office injection of Botox A targeting the lateral cricoarytenoid (LCA) muscle can be a safe and effective treatment even for recurrent granulomas. In an earlier study Pham *et al.* (2012) showed complete resolution of granulomas in 2–8 weeks after treatment with thyroarytenoid Botox injections which compared very favourably to PPI therapy alone.

Laryngeal dysplasia/leukoplakia/hyperkeratosis

The above appear as irregular, white lesions on the vocal folds caused by an increase in keratin. The lesions may be small and isolated, cover much of the surface of the vocal folds and may be accompanied by inflammation and generalised oedema. Consequently, the mucosal wave may be minimally affected by a small lesion, or be absent or disturbed by a more extensive lesion. Hyperkeratosis is precipitated by irritants to the vocal tract, allergies, chronic inflammation or radiation and results in a very low-pitched and rough voice. Karatayli-Ozgursoy *et al.* (2015) conducted a single-institution review over 20 years and noted that overall progression of laryngeal dysplasia to cancer had remained stable at a rate of approximately 8%. They suggest that although laryngeal dysplasia remains a disease predominantly found in males with a mean age at diagnosis of approximately 68 years, they noted demographic changes towards diagnosis at earlier ages. Treatment includes radiotherapy, increased use of microflap excision techniques, laser treatment, along with therapy to reduce irritants and vocal misuse, encouraging vocal hygiene and establishing a voice adequate for the needs of the patient are all options. Isenberg *et al.* (2008) found that the risk of developing malignancy appears to correlate with the severity of dysplasia present on initial biopsy.

Laryngeal papilloma

Laryngeal papilloma involves benign epithelial tumours caused by infection with the human papilloma virus (HPV). They are the most common benign neoplasms affecting the larynx and upper respiratory tract in both children and adults.

However, although papilloma may resolve spontaneously, they can be life-threatening because of airway obstruction from growth and proliferation of the papilloma lesions (Andrus and Shapshay, 2006) and may result, very occasionally, in the need for tracheostomy or even laryngectomy. Immediate post-operative results indicate that microdebriding is as safe as CO_2 laser (Pasquale *et al.*, 2009). In instances of repeated microsurgical intervention, thin vocal folds, scarring and long-standing dysphonia may result.

Depending on the extent of the papilloma, there may be variable disturbance to the mucosal wave and mild to severe dysphonia or aphonia.

Laryngeal web

Tewfik (2011) describes the condition as follows: 'Incomplete recanalization of the laryngotracheal tube during the third month of gestation leads to different degrees of laryngeal webs. Laryngeal webs may manifest with symptoms ranging from mild dysphonia to significant airway obstruction depending on the size of the web. Stridor is rare in patients who have a posterior interarytenoidal web.'

When there is a congenital laryngeal web, a disorder of voice may have been present since childhood, with little response to episodes of voice therapy due to the structural abnormality. Usually the laryngeal web is anteriorly in the vocal folds and forms a web at the anterior commissure, thus inhibiting normal movement during vibration and limiting the mucosal wave. Voice is often high-pitched and breathy with little intonation possible and may involve stridor. The treatment of choice may be surgical intervention, depending on the site and extent of the web, with laser surgery as a preference to avoid regrowth. A laryngeal web may also result from laryngeal trauma or from surgery where bilateral vocal fold surgery has been necessary and adhesions have formed as a web.

Sub-mucous haemorrhages

Vocal fold sub-mucous haemorrhages occur when there is rupture of blood vessels due to phonotrauma and extreme effort in voicing. There is bleeding into the superficial layer of the lamina propria. They may be seen as a small mass on the free edge of the vocal fold and may vary in size and site of injury. The mucosal wave may be limited in the affected area of the vocal fold or observed as reduced amplitude of vibration in the affected vocal fold. The patient often experiences a sudden disturbance to voice. This should be treated by voice rest to allow healing and recovery in the vocal fold. All habitual or recurring factors of extreme vocal effort should be addressed and any MTD should be treated to avoid recurrence. Occasionally the haemorrhage may become encapsulated into a cyst or polyp. This usually resolves spontaneously with time, but may require eventual surgical removal. Lucian Sulica at the Sean Parker Institute for the Voice, Weill Cornell Medicine (voice.weill.cornell.edu) notes the difference between the treatment of voice rest for a single, isolated haemorrhage as compared to repeated haemorrhage where there is an underlying cause, be it related to harmful voice behaviour or some other aetiology. In repeated haemorrhage, delicate microlaryngoscopy may be required to remove or repair any small irregularities or blood vessels prone to bleeding.

Sulcus vocalis

The two main types of pathological sulci are sulcus vergeture and sulcus vocalis where there occurs structural malformation of the vocal fold ranging from minor invagination to deep focal pits. Sulcus vergeture or Type 2 sulcus are a less common disorder, or less commonly diagnosed, involving an atrophic groove under the free edge of the vocal fold, while Type 3 sulci or sulcus vocalis manifests as an open cyst pocket lined with thick epithelium which goes as deep as the vocal ligament or muscle. Colton *et al.* (2011) suggest it may be difficult to distinguish these two forms of sulcus and indeed they may only become clear during microsurgery. It causes harsh, breathy dysphonia or may be asymptomatic and appear as increased stiffness of the vocal folds, a spindle-shaped gap in closure and reduced mucosal wave. Treatment options prior to considering surgery should involve the reduction of all known sources of mechanical trauma. Surgery is not a guarantor of success as scarring can occur, resulting in stiffness of the vocal fold and subsequent dysphonia. Therapy needs to be tailored to each patient, as a single treatment modality will not work in all cases. Whatever the surgery, most patients have supplementary injection laryngoplasty of the vocal fold.

Post-radiotherapy

Following radiotherapy for carcinoma of the larynx, the voice may be low-pitched and rough due to the side effects of the treatment. Bibby *et al.* (2007) report that at 12 months post-treatment, side effects may include vocal fold scarring, atrophy, and/or fibrosis, with the effects of these having possible negative effects on the voice in ways similar to the effects of the cancer itself. Depending on the extent and site of the lesion which has been treated, there may be disturbance to the mucosal wave because of the vocal fold stiffness. It is advisable for patients undergoing radiotherapy to be informed about reduction and avoidance of vocal effort, as dysphonia may occur with variable severity during and after radiotherapy, as may dysphagia. Patients should be advised regarding reduction of irritants, reduction in voice misuse, and establishing good voice techniques to minimise disturbance and achieve optimal recovery of voice. Van Gogh *et al.* (2012) conducted a study to assess the long-term effects of voice therapy treatment versus no treatment. After 13 months results showed that voice therapy was not just a short-lived improvement but may result in a better voice for a period of at least one year. More long-term randomised controlled trials are needed.

Tuomi *et al.* (2014) noted general improvement in voice and self-assessment of voice function after completion of radiotherapy. General improvement was seen for both a control and a study group in terms of vocal fatigue and vocal loudness but no change in vocal hoarseness. Results suggested positive effects of voice rehabilitation in both quality and self-perceived function.

Traumatic injury/scarring of the vocal folds

Scarring may be the result of traumatic injury, repeated surgery, inflammatory, neoplastic, congenital or other causes (Neuenschwander *et al.*, 2001). It may lead to scarring of the mucosa and stiffness of the vocal folds, resulting in disturbance or absence of the mucosal wave in the most affected vocal fold and rough, breathy voice. Scarring can range from mild to severe and can occur in one spot or along the full length of the vocal fold – the degree of scarring correlates with the degree of voice problems due to the varying degrees of loss of ability of the vocal fold to vibrate. In addition, those patients who due to improved resuscitation techniques survive serious road traffic accidents, attempted suicides or assaults may likely present with scarring of the vocal folds.

Although therapy aims to reduce all excess effort and facilitate optimal voice production, the prognosis for full recovery of voice will be limited by the extent and type of scarring. The scar tissue alters the viscoelasticity of the vocal fold and as the scar is in fact 'disorganised tissue' in the vibratory layer of the vocal fold it affects the resulting vocal quality (The

Voice Foundation website, www.voicefoundation.org). The use of a polymer such as hyaluronic acid for the treatment of vocal fold scars was explored a decade ago (Chhetri and Mendelsohn, 2010) and showed promise as a form of replacement therapy. More recently, Tateya *et al.* (2015) suggested that understanding the homeostasis of HA in scarred vocal fold tissue should enable new and better treatments for vocal fold scarring. More recent developments have looked at results from adipose derived stromal vascular fraction (SVF) as a possible treatment option in vocal fold scarring (Mattei *et al.*, 2017) but further studies are needed. The extracellular matrix properties of an injection of mesenchymal stem cells (MSCs) are also proving positive.

Organic voice disorders - neurological

Vocal fold paralysis/paresis

The external branch of the superior laryngeal nerve provides the motor supply to the cricothyroid muscle, with the 10th cranial nerve, the vagus, supplying the remaining laryngeal muscles. Due to the course of the vagus nerve, the left branch is more liable to injury than the right, with ensuing disturbance to vocal fold activity. Any damage or disturbance to the innervation of the intrinsic muscles of the larynx has the potential for vocal fold paralysis. This may be transient or permanent, complete or incomplete, and patients are normally advised that recovery can continue for a year after the trauma. Patients often describe a sudden loss of voice quality and power. This may be associated with an illness as innocuous as influenza or may follow surgical intervention, for example, thyroidectomy, coronary artery bypass grafting or endarterectomy.

Vocal fold paresis and paralysis comprise a range from mild to severe of abnormal laryngeal muscle function. Paresis can easily be missed as the patient may experience only a very mild vocal fatigue at the end of the day. On videostroboscopy, the affected fold will be seen to be lacking in tension and to have no mucosal wave. The position of the vocal fold may vary. If the paralysed fold is fixed in the paramedian position (in adduction), respiration may be disturbed but voice may be only slightly impaired. In bilateral adductor paralysis, there may be severe dyspnoea but almost normal phonation. Conversely, if the paralysis results in the intermediate position, the effects on voice are profound, with phonatory loss, breathy voice and disturbance of normal breathing patterns during attempted phonation. In vocal fold paralysis normal coughing may be disturbed. There may be a reduction in contact and glottal closure and some patients may report a degree of dysphagia.

Paralysis or paresis of the vocal folds may resolve spontaneously during the first year. However, given the potential for excessive effort by the patient in an attempt to phonate fully, recovery may be greatly enhanced by therapeutic intervention and, for example, bulk injection within this period, to avoid any MTD (Schindler *et al.*, 2008).

In some instances the most favourable results for the treatment of mild to moderate glottic insufficiency will be achieved by bulk injections to the vocal fold (Mallur and Rosen, 2010). Laryngeal framework surgery, however, can change the position and tension of the vocal folds safely without direct surgical intervention in the vocal fold proper. Many years of experience with phonosurgery have proved its usefulness in treating dysphonia related to unilateral vocal fold paralysis, vocal fold atrophy and pitch-related dysphonias. Emerging treatments have focused on neuromodulation, reinnervation, laryngeal pacing, gene therapy and stem cell therapy. While these approaches have promising potential, the evidence of success is limited and more clinical trials are needed before conclusions may be drawn.

However, although there may be instant improvement associated with these techniques, they should always be in partnership with therapeutic assessment and advice to maximise improvement and minimise a secondary MTD.

Spasmodic adductor dysphonia

Spasmodic adductor dysphonia is thought to be neurological in origin. The vocal folds and the supraglottic region are extremely compressed, with voice being produced on little out-going airflow and with possible explosions of normal voice as the laryngeal muscles relax intermittently. Vegetative and reflexive functions are normal. On videostroboscopy the mucosal wave is absent during phonation. Voice, however, may be quite normal for some activities such as reading, reciting or singing, but is disturbed in spontaneous speech and often described as strained strangled voice. Adductor spasmodic dysphonia is the most common type with 85–90% of the cases. Treatment is generally laryngeal injection of Botox, which is temporary but will last about three months. Dose-dependent Type A Botox is usually injected in both sides for Adductor Spasmodic Dysphonia; however, for Abductor Spasmodic Dysphonia the Botox dose is usually one-sided. Some side effects may occur, such as difficulty swallowing. Therapeutic intervention is thought to be inadequate as the sole treatment. Generally it is best treated by injection of *Botulinum* toxin (Botox) to effect a reduction in muscle spasm. Initially this may result in some dysphagia, but this should resolve within a short space of time with normal phonation and comfort. The injection may be helpful over a period of six months, but is not always a curative measure as repeated injections may be required. The multifactorial aetiology of spasmodic dysphonia may also lead to predisposing and perpetuating factors, for example, the irritation of GORD or LPR, psychological stress or conflict.

Spasmodic abductor dysphonia

This is less common than Spasmodic Adductor Dysphonia. It involves the sudden contraction of the posterior cricoarytenoid muscles, which causes the vocal folds to abduct and results in breathy and weak voice. Botox is injected into the affected muscles, usually on only one side to reduce the spasmodic activity.

Mixed spasmodic adductor/abductor dysphonia

Some experts report a mixed form of the disorder which is not common and which requires careful and accurate diagnosis at a specialised clinic to determine the best placement of Botox injection.

Bowing of the vocal folds

Neurological disorders may often present initially as weakness of voice and reduction in vocal muscle tension with or without bowing of the vocal folds. It is the experience of the author that patients with Parkinson's disease also frequently present with ventricular fold hyperadduction due to vocal fold inadequacy for the required phonatory environment (Belafsky *et al.*, 2002). Clinicians must, therefore, assess the patient as fully as possible to discover any abnormality in respiration, vocal fold movement, tongue, soft palate, lip or facial movement and/or dysphagia because several neurological disorders present with similar symptoms. Patients may feel well in other respects but may exhibit minimal signs of tremor in any of the muscles described above or present with reduced facial expression.

Where it is known that the patient has suffered a cerebrovascular incident and presents with dysarthria, associated respiratory and phonatory dysfunction may be present with bowing of the vocal folds and loss of tension. Just as it is possible to facilitate improvement in dysarthria with a course of therapy, so it may be possible to enable some restoration of function of respiration and phonation within the limits of the patient's general improvement.

Neurological disease

A voice disorder may be one of the few symptoms noted by patients in the early stages of progressive neurological disease, especially in Parkinson's disease (Sidor, 2010). Many experienced clinicians will also report patient referrals which present in the early stages as dysphonia only, and subsequently are diagnosed as a progressive neurological condition such as Parkinson's disease, myasthenia gravis or motor neurone disease (MND). Patients may also present with changes in nasal resonance, articulation or dysphagia. The assessment and diagnosis of the progressive disorder is vital to good patient management and determining the best treatment options. It is a given that for some patients with a neurological impairment such as MND, frequency of exercise, for example, in intensive articulation therapy may be disadvantageous as the increased muscle fatigue may in turn lead to an increase in the presenting symptoms. With Parkinson's disease there are currently two different types of SLT intervention available in the UK: standard National Health Service (NHS) speech and language therapy and Lee Silverman Voice Treatment (LSVT; Ramig *et al.*, 2001), a more intensive therapy which looks at increasing vocal loudness. It is not completely clear if one or both of these treatments is effective or acceptable to people with Parkinson's disease. A large scale multi-centred randomised controlled trial is currently underway in the UK (PD COMM; Sackley *et al.*, 2018). This trial, the findings of which are due in mid 2022, is looking at whether there is a benefit in Lee Silverman Voice Treatment versus standard speech and language therapy versus control in Parkinson's disease (pilot feasibility studies: biomedcentral.com.2018).

Along with personal choice, it is important to note that patients who are at the centre of a person-centred care pathway may wish for a different outcome to that of, for example, vocal loudness, as is the target in LSVT Loud™. It is important to always carefully review the patient's preferred outcomes on an ongoing basis and as always their wishes must be part of the future and current treatment dialogue. For those clinicians working within a Solution-Focused Brief Therapy (SFBT) framework, loudness may not be part of the patient's equation.

Progressive neurological disorders require specialised clinicians to assess and advise according to the stage in the disorder that the patient presents. Knowledge and expertise of Alternative and Augmentative Communication (AAC) equipment and voice/message banking are important tools for the clinician. An additional consideration are the logistical aspects of attendance; it may be very difficult for patients to attend regularly, let alone more than once a week, when intensive therapy is to be provided.

Benign essential tremor

Benign essential tremor results in tremor in the voice which may be mistaken for early signs of Parkinson's disease or other neurological disorders. This tremor, however, is benign and not indicative of progressive neurological disease, but must be diagnosed by a suitably qualified clinician. The entire larynx may be observed to tremor rhythmically, resulting in a shaky voice quality. It is generally associated with elderly patients, but can be diagnosed in younger people too. Sidor (2010) notes that it is most common in its presentation in the second and sixth decade of life. It can be responsive to voice therapy to reduce tension and facilitate optimal voice production techniques.

Head and neck cancer

It is not within the scope of this book or the knowledge of the author to focus on the Head and Neck specialty. There are many articles and specialist books which do so with expertise and rigour, but a brief comment is made here regarding the intervention of the clinician at different periods in the treatment journey.

Although any head and neck tumour may result in changes to voice production and voice quality, the primary and initial concern for the Head and Neck Team is the health of the patient and the best options for treatment or surgery. The voice clinician, as an essential part of this team, is involved throughout the patient journey, but may be more involved initially in swallowing advice and therapy rather than in the voice disorder. As with many of the disorders discussed, the first aim is to avoid a MTD as the patient attempts to compensate for vocal inadequacy. Further to that, the discussion on treatment options must focus on the specifics of the patient's treatment, surgery and general management and is therefore unique to each patient.

Summary

Although the disorders and vocal fold conditions discussed in this chapter appear clear when presented in text form, patients rarely completely conform to these descriptions and may present with multiple or mixed disorders. It is therefore essential that all aspects of the disorder are considered and that clinicians follow professional guidelines in waiting for an accurate diagnosis of the vocal fold condition before beginning treatment of any patient.

A summary of each disorder follows in Table 3.1, with vocal symptoms, videostroboscopic appearance, vocal fold appearance and suggestions for intervention and potential medicosurgical decisions. Every effort has been made to make sure that all surgical and treatment options are current, but it should be noted that developments in phonomicrosurgery are growing at pace, so regrettably it may be that some may be superseded within a short space of time. As ever, clinicians are encouraged to seek further guidance from team members and expert colleagues in the field, particularly if there are any concerns that are not addressed through discussion and multidisciplinary team working.

Table 3.1 Voice disorders summary chart

Condition	Vocal symptoms	Videostroboscopy	Vocal fold appearance	Mucosal wave	Intervention
Functional Voice disorders – MTD					
Posterior glottic chink	Breathy, sometimes with excess effort and possible hypertonicity	Lack of approximation posteriorly in the vocal folds	Possible stiffness	Reduced mucosal wave	Resolve precipitating and perpetuating factors and inadequacies of voice technique
Lateral constriction/ hyperadduction	Tense and forced quality of voice – voice fatigue may be present	Lateral constriction – vocal folds and possibly supraglottic muscles contract in a 'squeezing' manner during phonation	Hypertonicity	The mucosal wave may be reduced due to muscle stiffness	Resolve precipitating and perpetuating factors, attention to voice technique, voice management and vocal loading
Antero-posterior contraction	Low-pitched voice, sometimes breathy, voice fatigue and increased effort	Raised laryngeal position, not always possible to view vocal folds due to reduced antero-posterior space	Contraction of vocal folds and supraglottic area antero-posteriorly	Reduced mucosal wave	Tension reduction in neck, larynx, lowering of laryngeal position, improved voice technique and pitch placement
Ventricular phonation	Low-pitched, forced and rough voice with possible diplophonia	Hypertrophy and/or hyperadduction of the ventricular folds during phonation	Vocal folds may not be visible	Vocal folds may not be visible	Strategies are linked to the aetiology
Bowing of the vocal folds	Breathy, weak voice with possible raised pitch	Poor approximation of the vocal folds and 'bowing' during phonation	Vocal folds are often thin, loss of elasticity	Poor mucosal wave	Strategies are linked to the aetiology
Psychogenic voice disorders					
Hyperadduction	Various manifestations: effortful, 'squeezed-out' voice, little/no outgoing airflow, ingressive airflow, normal phonation intermittent with disorder	Normal laryngeal appearance at rest and vegetative functions, vocal folds and possibly the supraglottic muscles contract and constrict during phonation	Hypertonicity	Reduced mucosal wave	Strategies are linked to the aetiology

(continued)

Table 3.1 (Cont.)

Condition	Vocal symptoms	Videostroboscopy	Vocal fold appearance	Mucosal wave	Intervention
Hyperabduction	Absence of phonation, whisper or no airflow, may be constant or intermittent	Normal laryngeal appearance at rest and vegetative functions, approximation of vocal folds is absent during phonation	Normal laryngeal appearance at rest	Absent	Strategies are linked to aetiology
Organic voice disorders – structural					
Laryngitis	Pitch may be lowered, breathy and/or rough voice quality, hyperfunctional voice possible	Stiffness and reduced amplitude of excursion of vocal folds during vibration	Possible thickening of vocal folds, oedema and/or some irregularity of the vocal fold free edge	Lack of mucosal wave	Address precipitating or perpetuating factors, inadequate and faulty voice production techniques, facilitate good voice management and reduce vocal demand. PPI therapy
Vocal nodules	Effortful voice, pitch and voice breaks, possible diplophonia, increasing symptoms with use	Often antero-posterior contraction and stiffness of vocal folds	Will vary according to unilateral or bilateral lesion and size/site of lesion	May be disturbance of the vibratory patterns and mucosal wave	Voice care, reduction of irritants and vocal demand, facilitate optimal voice production technique, good voice management; may spontaneously resolve with therapeutic intervention or may require surgical intervention; best results may be combination of therapy and microsurgery
Vocal fold polyps	Voice is rough, breathy, often with pitch and voice breaks and diplophonia	Disturbance to vocal fold movement may be great or insignificant depending on the site of the lesion	Variable presentation	Variable presentation	Combination of surgery and therapeutic intervention, voice care, reduction of irritants, eradicate vocal misuse, facilitate adequate voice production
Vocal fold cysts	Voice may be unaffected or effortful, breathy, with pitch and voice breaks	Cysts usually unilateral and similar in appearance to vocal nodules or polyps	Increased stiffness in the vocal fold	Absence of the mucosal wave in the affected fold	Combination of surgical and therapeutic intervention

Oedema	Voice varies according to the extent of the lesion, often low-pitched and effortful, may be breathy	Oedema may be unilateral or bilateral, minimal or widespread across the vocal fold surface	Vocal fold thickening and stiffness in affected area	Poor or absent mucosal wave in affected area	Possible surgical intervention dependent on the extent of the oedema, possible reduction with advice and therapy: voice care, reduction of irritants and misuse, facilitation of optimal voice production techniques
Reinke's oedema	Low-pitched, effortful, breathy and rough voice	Affected area appears to flap rather than vibrate	May be unilateral or bilateral, gelatinous appearance of the affected area of vocal folds	No mucosal wave in affected area	Treat causative factors – surgical and therapeutic intervention may be combined, facilitate optimal voice care and voice production
Contact ulcer	Sometimes 'creaky' voice, fatigue and pain – dysphonia may vary from no voice disturbance to continuous	May be unilateral or bilateral	Vocal folds may be thickened	Mucosal wave may be unaffected	Varies according to aetiology, may involve surgical and therapeutic intervention, reduction in MTD, voice care, the establishment of adequate voice production. PPI therapy
Granuloma	May be sudden onset, breathy, low-pitched, possibly rough voice or no voice disturbance	May be little or no disturbance to vocal fold movement	Usually on the vocal process, may become large, with a corresponding groove on the opposing vocal fold	May be little or no disturbance to mucosal wave	Treatment of LPR, reduction in irritants, voice intervention; facilitate optimal voice production and reduce MTD symptoms; surgical intervention may be required. Botox Type A injections to temporarily limit vocal fold mobility

(continued)

Table 3.1 (Cont.)

Condition	Vocal symptoms	Videostroboscopy	Vocal fold appearance	Mucosal wave	Intervention
Laryngeal dysplasia/ leukoplakia/ hyperkeratosis	Disturbance to voice may vary from minimal or non-existent to low-pitched, rough and weak voice	Varies according to the degree of the lesion	Varies from small lesions to widespread, unilateral or bilateral	Disturbance to mucosal wave varies according to the extent of the lesion	Surgical and therapeutic intervention often combined, attention to voice care and reduction in MTD
Laryngeal papilloma	Variable disturbance to voice from none to severe	Varies according to the degree and site of the lesion	Wart-like growths which may be on the free edge of the vocal folds or extend to the whole larynx and varies according to the degree and site of the lesion	Varies according to the degree and site of the lesion	Microdebriding, repeated surgery may result in thin and scarred vocal folds – therapy facilitates optimal voice production within the confines of the recovery or recurrence of the lesion
Laryngeal web	Voice is often high-pitched, breathy, weak, with little variation possible – there may be stridor	Usually the web is at the anterior end of the vocal folds and inhibits vocal fold movement	The web is visible between the vocal folds	Mucosal wave is inhibited by the web	Surgical intervention is usually necessary, combined with therapy; facilitate optimal voice production and quality; prognosis varies
Sub-mucous haemorrhages	May be sudden disturbance to voice quality following the instance of voice trauma	Small mass on the free edge of the vocal fold, will vary in size and site	Haemorrhage is visible on the vocal fold	Mucosal wave is limited in the area of the lesion	Voice rest facilitates healing and recovery, voice care reduction in voice misuse factors, attention to any MTD, may require surgical intervention
Sulcus vocalis	May be asymptomatic or breathy, harsh voice	Incomplete closure with a spindle-shaped gap between the vocal folds	Usually bilateral groove in medial margin of the longitudinal surface of the vocal folds	Reduced mucosal wave	Microsurgery, therapy to reduce mechanical trauma, optimal voice production and voice care
Post-radiotherapy	Low-pitched, rough voice with possible increased effort on phonation	Vocal folds may be inflamed, dry and stiff	Vocal folds may be inflamed, dry and stiff, with possible hypertonicity due to increased effort	Possibly reduced mucosal wave	Voice care especially reduction of irritants, reduction of MTD, facilitate optimal voice production

Organic voice disorders – neurological

Vocal fold paralysis	Low-pitched, breathy, weak voice, little flexibility or stamina, possible pitch and voice breaks, possible respiratory disturbance, difficulty in sustained phonation; it may be transient, long-standing, permanent, minimal, moderate or severe	May be unilateral or bilateral, the affected vocal fold lacks tension and the arytenoid cartilage may prolapse	Mucosal wave is absent in the affected vocal fold	Therapy to reduce excess effort, facilitate optimal voice production within viable limits, bulk injection – if surgical intervention required, various surgical options are possible combined with therapeutic intervention as optimal approach
Spasmodic adductor dysphonia	Little outgoing airflow, compressed voice, possible 'explosions' of voice, may be normal voice quality in reading, reciting or spontaneous speech	During attempted phonation, there is compressions and constriction within the larynx and supraglottic area	Normal appearance and movement at rest and during vegetative functions or spontaneous speech	Botox (*Botulinum* toxin) injections to reduce muscle spasm in the affected muscles
Spasmodic abductor dysphonia	Breathy, weak voice	Vocal folds lack tension and approximation	May be present and normal within spontaneous phonation	Botox injection into the cricoarytenoid muscles
Bowing of the vocal folds	Breathy, weak voice with possible raised pitch	Poor approximation of the vocal folds and 'bowing' during phonation	Poor mucosal wave	Strategies are linked to the aetiology
Neurological disease	Varies according to the disorder	Vocal folds may appear 'bowed' during voice	Poor mucosal wave	Varies according to the disorder
Benign essential tremor	Voice may be weak and breathy, tremor in pitch and general voice production parameters	Varies according to the disorder	Varies according to the disorder	Voice care, reduce any MTD and facilitate optimal voice production techniques

Head and neck cancer

Tumour	Varies according to the disorder	Entire larynx may be seen to tremor rhythmically	May appear lacking in tension	May be absent
		Varies according to the disorder	Varies according to the disorder	Varies according to the disorder

BUILDING THE PATIENT PROFILE

Introduction

Building the patient profile is a gradual and careful process. It provides the clinician with a full understanding of the predisposing, precipitating and perpetuating factors which have impacted the patient. This then informs the decision-making process and shapes future treatment and management.

The first contact

It is always important to consider the various thoughts and emotions that many voice patients experience when they attend their first appointment, involving apprehension, fear, scepticism and even hostility, which can arise out of accurate as well as inaccurate information. While the internet is helpful in so many respects, it also can furnish patients with unreasonable expectations and misinformation, particularly where the patient has no background knowledge to help in filtering the online information. Furthermore, some patients, despite previous discussions with their General Practitioner and Ear, Nose and Throat consultant, are still unsure of the reason for referral to voice therapy and can be uncertain as to why they have to attend the SLT clinic, what to expect from the session and what will be expected of them during the consultation. It is extremely helpful to forward an information pack to the patient prior to the first appointment, giving details of what will take place at the appointment and who will be present. This can either be a hard copy for those who do not have internet access, or an online file attachment.

Clinical practice changes from centre to centre but in some clinics the practice is to send out the appointment letter with an information leaflet and possibly a questionnaire for the patient to complete and bring on their first attendance. There are many different questionnaires suitable for this purpose, which focus on different aspects of information gathering. For example, the Vocal Performance Questionnaire (VPQ; Carding *et al.*, 1999) focuses on self-reported information regarding the patient's perception of their voice quality and how it affects their life. The Voice Severity Scale (VOISS; Deary *et al.*, 2003) gives a self-reported rating on the severity of the disorder. The Voice Handicap Index-10 (VHI-10) and the VPQ are similar, short, convenient, internally consistent, uni-dimensional tools giving good overall indicators of the severity of voice disorders. These measures have high validity, the best reported reliability to date, good sensitivity to change and excellent utility ratings. These instruments are therefore likely to provide high-quality outcome information irrespective of whether the treatment choice is phonosurgery, voice therapy, pharmacological therapy or a combination of several approaches.

As has already been noted, clinical assessment and therapeutic intervention choices are highly personal and are dependent on a number of variables. For the author the use of the Voice Impact Profile (VIP; Martin and Lockhart, 2005) has proved highly effective over many years. The VIP uses information garnered from the questionnaire, which takes 10–15 minutes to complete, to provide foundational case history details and then uses the resultant information to guide decision making in terms of future intervention. The VIP questionnaire and interactive disc produce a profile which is a visual representation of the patient's responses. The profile provides a valuable background for discussion at the next individual contact with the patient, giving feedback or seeking further information where needed. It provides visual feedback, which the findings of Chan *et al.* (2002) and Makdessian *et al.* (2004) support, that providing written materials to patients post-consultation has a significant, positive influence upon subsequent recall of clinical information/advice. This process facilitates discussion and explanations of the ten different sections of the VIP and the potential for negative impact on voice. The sections are: General Health, Vocal History, Vocal Health, Vocal Care, Vocal Demand, Vocal Status, Voice Geneogram, Anxiety and Stress, Social Functioning and Environment. This chapter will follow the outline of the VIP and look at the way in which the range and diversity of the information gained from each section will contribute to building the patient profile and in turn underpin the decision-making process that will shape future intervention for the individual.

While individual first contact sessions were at one time the 'norm' when working with voice patients, increasing numbers of referrals, increasing waiting times and unchanging clinical capacity has led to a rethink of this approach and research (Lockhart, 2011; Law *et al.*, 2012; Almeida *et al.*, 2015; Burt and Fletcher, 2019) has suggested that clinical efficiency and effectiveness may well be increased if the first contact for patients is at a Voice Information Group, which can involve up to a maximum of 12 patients in one group. Clinicians will adopt their own format and content, but an example of a Voice Information Group that ran very successfully in Lanarkshire is outlined here. The group involved a specialist therapist and an assistant, with the group receiving information on the normal larynx and voice produc-tion, vocal misuse factors, voice care, voice management and voice therapy. Visual teaching resources illustrated how the larynx and vocal folds may change in appearance and function when excess muscle tension creates hyperfunction, sometimes progressing to a muscle tension dysphonia (MTD) and possible secondary pathology. Towards the end of the group session and after being offered the potential of one-to-one discussion, patients were asked to decide whether they wished to apply the advice given and also attend for therapy, apply the advice given and return for an individual review appointment in 3–4 months, or apply the advice and be discharged. Clinical audit of this group (Lockhart, 2011) showed positive outcome results and will be discussed further in Chapter 8.

It is not the job of the clinician to use this first visit to 'sell' the voice package of assessment and therapeutic intervention. Indeed, the experience of many clinicians is that persuading reluctant patients to attend often results in their eventual failure to attend. It is therefore much more effective to provide as much information as possible, with the patient taking full responsibility for opting in or out of therapy.

Far removed from the paternalistic model of treatment, shared decision making and self-management support is changing patient care models (Ahmed *et al.*, 2014). Across the four countries of the UK, the vision of person- or patient-centred health care has emerged in recent years as a major theme in health policy. The trend, at least rhetorically, has been towards seeing people as active partners in, rather than simply passive recipients of, health care. Despite the often used language of 'patient-centred' care, acknowledgement of the contribution that families and wider social networks make to both health and the provision of health care has also been recognised. Family carers in particular are increasingly identified as a group with whom professionals and services should collaborate to ensure a more joined-up approach to care across formal and informal settings. Prior to the Voice Impact Profile becoming the author's standard procedure as the first contact, it proved difficult to collect all the necessary information in one visit and the initial interview and case history often took more than one session. It is the author's opinion that this difficulty is largely addressed by using the VIP and, if possible, a Voice Information Group. Depending on the patient's choice as to whether to return for an individual review or to attend for a course of therapy, there is the opportunity for further discussion and information gathering to supplement the existing case-history information before therapy commences.

It should be noted, however, that some patients experience difficulty in supplying information for various reasons and are unable to complete a questionnaire or to self-report. For example, patients may have visual impairment, illiteracy, dyslexia, mental health issues, poor concentration, or English may not be their first language. Certainly, someone may complete the VIP on behalf of the patient, but if information has to be sourced from family members or friends, it may lead to bias and/or potentially critical issues being overlooked. Asking sensitive questions with a family member translating may compromise the veracity of the response and so, if possible, it is best to use the services of a translator. In that way the clinician is assured of a response devoid of any emotional 'overlay', confusion or coercion. With an experienced clinician using a relaxed, conversational approach, the relevant information and detail can be gained through individual contact.

As an observer, watching a skilled clinician 'chat' and ask open-ended questions, free from cultural, ethnic or racial bias, relating to different aspects of the patient's history, can seem a simple task. Many students, however, will report the difficulties experienced in this approach and the tendency to lose focus and time on irrelevancies. Paradoxically, this style of interviewing is probably the most expert of all, for it enables the patient to relax and be at ease in giving personal information without the sense of interrogation, while the clinician probes to unearth the most relevant details. When observing the experienced clinician, one notes that the conversation is subtly directed along certain avenues. The information gained from the patient is balanced by some explanation to aid understanding of the nature and progression of the disorder, the ultimate planning of treatment and the prognosis for recovery. This process of open questioning, restatement and summarising for clarification, of obtaining information from the perspective of the individual patient and others in his or her environment is a critical skill, usually honed over many years. In this way important factors can be identified while the patient is encouraged and informed, both of which may resolve some of the initial reticence and scepticism. Studies of medical consultation indicate that what patients value is warmth, care, concern and the ability to explain clearly. Patient recall and understanding is enhanced when simple, clear and well-structured explanations are provided. Improved recall and understanding according to Brown et al. (2006), lead to higher patient satisfaction and higher patient compliance, and ultimately contribute to health improvement.

The author makes no apology in citing the words of Aronson (1985), which are as pertinent today as they were 35 years ago:

> Any in-depth study of voice disorders forces us to conclude that so long as clinicians obtain privileged information from patients; so long as people have voice problems because of life stress and interpersonal conflict; so long as voice disorders produce anxiety, depression, embarrassment and self-consciousness; so long as patients need a sympathetic person with whom they can discuss their distress will speech pathologists need to consider their training incomplete until they have learned the basic skills of psychological interviewing and counseling.

Other styles of case-history taking may include checklists or clinic proformas, of which there are many, as well as standardised assessment procedures and questionnaires. All of these have value, and clinicians have many options in an interview situation, choosing the most relevant tools for each patient, while maintaining an awareness of equality and diversity factors. The clinician must therefore decide on the format of the first contact, the documentation and the style of interviewing. However, whatever format or questionnaires are used, it is important that certain goals are achieved during the first visit.

Whether it takes place in a group or individually, there must be opportunity for concerns to be raised, information exchanged and misconceptions addressed. Surprisingly, this process can often be aided by a group situation where the patient may feel less vulnerable due to the presence of others with similar difficulties. Patients may have had anecdotal information supplied to them by friends and family regarding their disorder, which can easily result in unnecessary anxiety and fear, due to lack of understanding and misinformation. The same lack of information can cause reluctance to comply or attend regularly. Time is required to discuss various options in therapy, enabling the patient to understand the 'cause and effect' relationship of attendance and non-attendance. While the patient must ultimately decide on the terms of the 'contract', it is the responsibility of the clinician to ensure that this decision is taken with the fullest possible knowledge, so that the patient moves along the health continuum from disorder back to health. It is worth recording at this point that Kessels (2003) reminds readers that on average a patient retains only a small amount of material. Patients' memory for medical information is often poor and inaccurate, especially when the patient is old or anxious. Bostrom (2006) reports that results from almost every aspect of listening measurements show that less than half of what is transmitted is retained, even within a few minutes. Patients tend to focus on diagnosis-related information and fail to register instructions on treatment. Simple and specific instructions are better recalled than general statements and changes in patient behaviour are unlikely to be sustained unless they are integrated in the cognitive structure of the patient/clinician relationship. Patients can be helped to remember medical information by use of explicit categorisation techniques. In addition, spoken information should be supported with written or visual material. Visual communication aids are especially effective in low-literacy patients, but it should not be assumed that a patient's ability to listen is correlated with other cognitive skills, as Bostrom (2006) suggests this is not the case, nor do video or multimedia techniques always improve memory performance or adherence to therapy.

A variety of interventions including written and recorded material, mind-maps, acronyms and cognitive approaches – such as the use of repetition of instructions, by both the clinician and the patient; summarisation of the session; giving advice in concrete and specific terms, and techniques to build confidence – could potentially influence how well patients can remember the advice given to them by the clinician. A very useful and still very pertinent systematic review of interventions to improve recall of medical advice in healthcare consultations (Watson and McKinstry, 2009) is recommended.

From the clinician's perspective, there must be an opportunity to gain insight into the patient's general motivation to change and to discuss appointment planning. The length of the care episode will be determined by a number of factors, for example the clinical setting, the prescribed number of sessions, the patient's personal situation, i.e. time lost from their work, increase in childcare cover or care of elderly relatives. Some clinics may be able to offer clinic appointments at flexible times to avoid loss of earnings or extra expenditure for patients. Similarly, it may be possible to consider intensive therapy over a short timescale, longer sessions at lengthy intervals and a number of different options. Ultimately, however, the therapy planning must be adapted to fit the patient's circumstances and needs, within the often limited resources of the service.

Documenting patient information

When documenting patient information, there will be a number of points to consider in line with the guidance offered by the Health and Care Professions Council (HCPC) and the Professional College with whom a clinician is registered. In the UK, the Royal College of Speech and Language has guidance to support members to adhere to the HCPC standards in the keeping of records, among which are policies on, for example:

- procedures for the creation, use, secure storage and appropriate sharing of records, in line with current legislation whatever context they work in and the periodic monitoring and reviewing of these procedures. Laws governing the length of time for case records to be stored vary from one authority to another, so clinicians need to be aware of the local policy for storage and disposal;
- ensuring that the records are fit for purpose, offer evidence of clear clinical reasoning and decision making, and are objective and concise. In addition, care records should be written promptly, as soon as practically possible after the activity occurred, signed and dated, using the date the service user was seen and the date the entry was made, if different;
- making chronological changes or corrections to care records clearly and self-identifying the care record entries, clearly identifying the service user throughout the record, according to local policy and practice;
- managing records according to all relevant legislation, guidance or policies – national and local, and ensuring that systems are in place for auditing records of work. It should be remembered that all notes represent a legal document and can be required for scrutiny in any case of audit, complaint or enquiry.

Biographical information

For some patients their past experiences of medical appointments will have prepared them to expect what can appear to be quite intrusive questioning. For some patients this is not a problem, but for others it can lead to a certain resistance to answer questions which seem to have little relevance or link to their medical condition. Indeed, it may be that information they gave to one professional has not been 'passed on' to the next professional who asks the same question. For that reason, before accessing biographical information it may be helpful to explain to the patient why there is a need to gather information on their home situation, the number of people living there and the relationships involved, through the lens of the voice disorder.

Obviously, in some homes, the interpersonal relationships can be complex and may be of great importance in contributing to the patient's disorder and the prognosis for recovery. At times it may be helpful to give examples of the impact of various activities on voice production, and the amount and type of voice usage which may adversely affect voice. For example, some households are very noisy with everyone habitually using raised voices simply to be heard. Where this happens, those involved may be quite unaware of the noise levels until attention is drawn to this.

The voice disorder

One of the difficulties associated with accurate reporting is the length of time that usually elapses between the patient noting the problem and actually seeing a clinician. Clinicians must, therefore, be particularly scrupulous in trying to elicit as much information as possible, recognising that reporting past events accurately is notoriously difficult. Describing voice quality is particularly difficult, even for the 'experts', so the use of a universal rating scale of voice quality is critical. Carding *et al.* (2009) recommend that routine voice outcome measurement should include an expert rating of voice quality such as the Grade–Roughness–Breathiness–Asthenia Strain scale (GRBAS; Hirano, 1981). The obvious limitation is that, in a clinical setting, expert rating of voice quality will probably be carried out by the treating clinician. Carding *et al.* go on to recommend to clinicians that the effect of clinical bias and the performance of less expert raters, if the clinician is working on their own, should not prevent clinicians from applying these measures in routine practice in order to determine the effectiveness of their treatments. It is worth remembering that with respect to voice quality ratings, clinician ratings may not always correlate with the patient's perceptions of their own voice quality scores.

It is often helpful if, in addition, the patient is encouraged to use a comparative scale such as higher/lower, louder/softer, more/less and to support this information with anecdotal evidence from family and friends. In this way, patients are encouraged to reflect more forensically on their voice quality, both how it sounds now and how it used to sound. Indeed, it can be useful to provide patients with examples of questions which they can ask friends, relations and colleagues. Examples of such questions could be: 'In your opinion is my voice higher, lower, more husky or less clear than it was?' Patient self-perception of vocal quality will be discussed more fully later in this chapter under Vocal Status.

General health

It is common for inexperienced clinicians or students to feel apprehensive when asking personal questions regarding health and medication, imagining that patients will be reticent or embarrassed to give this information. However, generally this is untrue. Patients are rarely reluctant to give information, especially if an explanation has been given regarding the relevance to the voice disorder and the confidentiality of the information gained. It can be helpful to use a proforma with headings on the course and recurrence of any illness and detailing previous or current medication. As in previous aspects of the case history, patients may be encouraged to talk, simply by asking them: 'Tell me about your health in general', 'Have you had any problems with ...?', 'What medication do you/did you take for that?'

Previous illness with details of surgery and/or hospitalisation

To ensure that any relevant physical illness is discussed, this all-encompassing heading should be included in the proforma. The clinician should not underestimate the relevance of an apparently unrelated illness or surgical procedure associated with the disturbance of respiration or phonation. For example, patients may report pain around the ribs following fracture of the ribs, a back injury, chest and/or heart surgery. They may then unconsciously restrict movement in that part of the body to avoid discomfort, not only during coughing or laughing but also during breathing for voice and speech. Similarly, back, neck, shoulder or chest pain may lead to a rigid posture and alteration in muscle habits for respiration and phonation. Weakness and fatigue after major illnesses can lead to respiration disturbance simply due to lack of energy, reduced muscle tension, low volumes of air and low airflow rate on phonation. These patterns may easily become habitual even when the original cause has resolved. It is also profitable to explore as fully as possible the emotional circumstances surrounding illness or surgery to ascertain any associated tension and anxiety, depression, adverse reaction of significant others, loss of status or loss of job, as well as the physical contributing factors.

Medication

Medication has been mentioned above and is obviously of great importance in the patient profile. Clinicians are encouraged to refer to articles and/or websites which detail the effects of medication in communication and voice, particularly as new pharmacological treatment regimens are introduced, sometimes with significant effects on the vocal fold mucosa and laryngeal physiology. For example, many websites note the possibility of side effects of voice disturbance from antidepressants, muscle relaxants, diuretics, antihypertensives (blood pressure medication), antihistamines (allergy medication) and anticholinergics (asthma medication). Commonly the side effect is dryness of the mucosal linings of the vocal tract and a dry, irritating cough, but there can be additional effects such as changes in coordination and proprioception, airflow, structure of the vocal folds and oedema, for example. Many patients now self-medicate, with 'over the counter' or 'online' medication, or favour the use of herbal remedies and/or vitamin supplements. They may be unaware of any side effects from these, including voice disturbance. Patients should always be encouraged to read the information provided on any medication, herbal or vitamin supplement especially if they are a frequent voice user in work or leisure activities. Similarly, the patient should be encouraged to disclose self-medication to the clinician. An additional caution should be delivered to older patients as there is a recognition that older people may respond quite differently, as an artefact of ageing, from younger patients who are taking the same medication.

Breathing

Any disturbance to respiration has the potential to change the phonatory system as air volumes and airflow control are key elements in normal voice. Similarly, any illness which involves such disturbance, whether short- or long-term, can result in residual respiratory muscle habits even after the illness has resolved. The common cold is probably one of the most frequent precipitators of voice disturbance when patients do not rest physically and vocally during the acute stage of irritation, congestion and/or increased secretions. The amount of vocal effort needed to produce acceptable voice is therefore increased with the possibility of a MTD being established. Similarly, various illnesses or surgical procedures may involve chest or back pain in the acute or post-operative period, with some patients reducing the amount of intercostal movement during respiration to reduce pain. This may result in inadequate support for phonation due to respiratory insufficiency.

Allergies

As noted, given the increase in 'over the counter' availability of medication, it is not uncommon for patients to self-diagnose and self-treat for many conditions, including allergies. The use of nasal sprays for hay fever or common nasal allergies may, in some cases, be very efficacious, but in others may become a habitual response to even slight nasal congestion with a negative impact on the nasal mucosa. Patients using sprays frequently for allergies should be encouraged to seek advice from their General Practitioner to ensure that the medication is appropriate and necessary. Patients suffering from recurring allergies may not only describe the obvious effect on the mucosa, the often copious secretions produced and the associated discomfort of constant watery eyes and runny nose, but may report some impact on the pharyngeal and laryngeal mucosa too, resulting in dysphonia (Dworkin *et al.*, 2009). In contrast, some patients diagnosed with allergies may be misdiagnosed as having LPR (Randhawa *et al.*, 2009; Roth and Ferguson, 2010) so it is important to explore this carefully.

Asthma and use of inhalers

Inhalers are now commonly prescribed for a variety of breathing difficulties and it is important that the clinician knows the length of time and frequency of usage of these. This is particularly so in the use of inhaled corticosteroids of which there are three main devices for inhalation therapy: pressurised metered-dose inhalers (MDIs), dry powder inhalers (DPIs) and soft-mist inhalers (SMIs) and it is important to know what type of inhaler the patient uses. Although inhaled steroids have few side effects, especially at lower doses, thrush (a yeast infection in the mouth) and hoarseness may occur, although this is rare. While it may be necessary for the patient to continue with this treatment, the impact of the medication is important to the prognosis and to the patient's understanding of contributing and perpetuating factors. A review of the patient's technique when using their inhaler is very important; for example, do they use a spacer as routine? Devices with metered-dose inhalers can help prevent side effects. Questions related to the patient's post-spray regime are similarly important, such as do they rinse their mouth and gargle after using their asthma inhaler? Encouraging patients to 'Rinse, gargle, swish and spit' is a good mantra. It should, however, be noted that the new-generation inhalers, where strictly measured amounts of corticosteroids are 'pre-delivered', have far reduced the previous likelihood of excessive amounts of corticosteroids reaching the vocal folds.

Back or joint pain

As discussed previously, any postural change may lead to altered respiration and laryngeal disturbance. It is also necessary to note the length and severity of any arthritic episode and the type of arthritis involved. For many patients, the wear and tear of life leads to changes in the spine and joints, and gradual alteration of posture and muscle movement. For others, rheumatoid arthritis may also affect the joints in and around the larynx. Again, it is important to note the medication prescribed and the potential side effects it may have on digestion, in irritating the digestive tract and causing reflux.

Digestion and diet

It is well recognised that reflux is of importance in the general condition of the vocal folds, as previously noted in Chapter 2. Any spillage of acid reflux into the larynx may result in irritation to, or inflammation of, the mucosal linings. Subsequent alteration in vibration characteristics and voice often leads to increased effort to overcome the hoarseness. Although some patients may be aware of digestive difficulty, this may not always be so and some patients have undiagnosed and untreated reflux until they are assessed by the voice clinician. Hiatus hernia may create similar reflux problems or intermittent pain leading to inhibited movement of the diaphragm. Various types of foods may be contributory factors in leading to thick saliva and dryness of the mouth. For instance, spicy foods may result in thirst and a dry mouth and while foods such as milk, cheese, and yogurt do not trigger the body to produce excess mucus, they can cause existing mucus to become thicker. With dryness of the mouth and thick secretions, it is likely that the patient will clear the throat more regularly to eliminate the tenacious secretions, resulting in irritation in the larynx. An additional consideration should be the possibility of a patient presenting with reflux as a result of unreported bulimia where patients experience digestive problems, including acid reflux and stomach pain. The sphincter controlling the oesophagus may become weaker, due to continued bouts of vomiting allowing acid to back up into the oesophagus and causing gastrointestinal symptoms. Anorexia may also cause voice quality changes, but those changes are more often the result of the effect of the process of starvation on most organ systems and the subsequent connection to anatomy, physiology, neuroanatomy and psychology than a direct effect on the vocal tract per se.

Smoking, alcohol, recreational drugs and caffeine

The negative effects of smoking are widely known and while it is not the role of the clinician to proselytise the anti-smoking message it is, however, helpful to discuss with the patient potential strategies for smoking reduction or cessation, or to suggest clinics, groups or treatments which are available locally. In any event, the patient should be encouraged as strongly as possible to be honest about the number of cigarettes or cigars smoked daily and should be encouraged to stop. This is particularly important in those conditions which are closely related to smoking, for example, Reinke's oedema. The patient must be made aware of the association and be encouraged to assume responsibility in this area, with the understanding that progress may be limited by continuing to smoke. Likewise the topic of recreational drugs should be raised because unfiltered marijuana smoke causes even greater irritation to the vocal tract than does tobacco. Information about patterns of cannabis consumption appears, to the author, to be relevant and reasonable to gather from patients with voice disorders. A recent systematic review (Meehan-Atrash *et al.*, 2019) of the effect of cannabis inhalation and voice disorders suggests that cannabis-only smoking is associated with changes in vocal fold appearance, respiratory symptoms and negative lung function changes, especially in heavy smokers. Results further suggest that cannabis smokers presenting with a voice disorder should undergo laryngeal imaging and complete pulmonary function testing when indicated and receive education about consumption methods and their association with voice disorders. Vaping, which had, at one stage, been advocated as safer than smoking, has been the subject of a report by The US Centres for Disease Control and Prevention (2020), advising that hundreds of e-cigarette users had been affected by lung injury; clinicians should therefore recommend that patients check online for up-to-date advice. Although patients may have an awareness of the relationship between cigarette smoking and cancer, there may be less awareness of the impact of heavy alcohol consumption on the voice. While patients may find the discussion of alcohol consumption a more sensitive issue than that of cigarette smoking, it should be addressed in an open manner with discussion of the negative effects of alcohol on the vocal folds in terms of dryness and irritation. When consumption of both alcohol and smoking is heavy, the risk of cancer is multiplied; 80% of throat and mouth cancer in men and 65% of throat and mouth cancer in women are linked to the combination of smoking and drinking (National Institute of Alcohol Abuse and Alcoholism, 2014, www.niaaa.nih.gov).

Chronic fatigue or recurring viral illness

Although there are many opinions on post-viral or chronic fatigue syndrome and similar illnesses, many clinicians have anecdotal details of patients suffering from such disorders with associated voice symptoms. While the differential diagnosis may pose some difficulties, it should not be too quickly labelled as a functional or psychosomatic disorder, but an accurate diagnosis should be pursued over time and supported by knowledge of the individual patient. In the author's experience, the variation in the severity of the illness may be mirrored by similar variation of voice quality.

Vocal history
The onset of the current disorder

Although it can be difficult for some patients to remember exact details of the onset of the disorder, most are prepared to be asked this question and have given it some thought. The patient may have only a rather vague impression of their voice deteriorating over a period of time, but even this is important as it signals that no specific incident may have occurred which involved sudden disturbance of voice. Where the onset is gradual, it is essential that the concomitant events, circumstances and health status before and around that time are explored. For example, common colds and flu are so often the precipitating factors leading to a gradual disturbance of voice quality. The patient may have had to fulfil normal daily duties before the irritation, inflammation and/or increased secretions of the upper respiratory tract have been resolved.

A sudden onset of dysphonia or aphonia does not automatically signal a psychogenic disorder. Traumatic injury to the vocal folds caused by excessive force or effort in voice or idiopathic vocal fold palsy may also lead to a sudden loss of voice. Because patients may not be aware of any contributing factors, the circumstances surrounding the onset must be explored as fully as possible. It can also be helpful to discuss the possibility that sudden onset can sometimes be stress-related, explaining the relationship between stress and muscular tension. On occasions, this may give patients 'permission' to admit to stress, often for the first time, feeling that they are in a situation where disclosure is acceptable. One must also note that anecdotal histories exist of patients diagnosed initially as having a psychogenic disorder only to find at later stages that a neurological condition or carcinoma existed. While these instances are rare, it is the thoroughness of the information gathering which brings us to the point of differential diagnosis.

The nature of the disorder (severity, duration and frequency)

The patient may need help to define the severity of voice disturbance at the onset and on all subsequent episodes. This may be achieved by using a scale of 1 to 10 in terms of severity, from normal to complete loss of voice. While this is subjective, it gives some information on the patient's perception. Similar to onset details, the severity and duration of each episode will help the clinician to determine the contributing and perpetuating factors, which may be keys to the aetiology. As with all subjective qualitative rating measures, it is important to carefully consider the patient's own personal definition of vocal quality, as their value judgement of their own voice is highly dependent on their own perceptual appreciation of vocal quality. A voice which the clinician, as the 'expert listener', may feel is very compromised in terms of vocal quality may not appear to be so to the patient. As in all other areas of clinical practice, the patient as the service user and, in turn, the expert on their own disorder needs to be carefully questioned as to the benchmark against which the rating is being assigned. For some patients a voice disorder is of little importance, their rating of 5 could be another's rating of 10.

The pattern of voice disturbance

The pattern of vocal change can be examined over any time frame, from a matter of hours of voice usage to the effect on voice over several months. Initially it may be helpful to ask open questions regarding patterns of disturbance, such as: 'When is your voice at its worst?', 'Does it vary at all?', 'Is there any pattern to the variation?', 'Does the voice deteriorate only when other factors are present, such as in dry or smoky atmospheres, in noisy conditions or when there is stress?', 'Are there other physical or emotional factors that occur along with the voice disorder?' For some, voice may deteriorate with what appears to be only a low-level demand, whereas others experience increased dysphonia only with high-level demand.

Previous episodes of voice therapy

While some information systems will give details of previous treatment episodes, it is important to discover from the patient any previous voice therapy or voice training, with as much detail as possible. The clinician should seek answers to the following questions:

- What were the circumstances of the referral?
- Who fulfilled the therapy?
- What did the therapy involve?
- Was the treatment episode completed?
- What was the outcome of therapy?
- Was the patient satisfied with the choice of therapy?
- What was the status of the patient when discharged from regular therapy?

Answers to all these questions are important factors in the management of the current episode, if the recurring pattern of dysphonia is to be addressed, resolved and patient compliance ensured.

Laryngeal examination

Professional guidelines will differ from country to country but in the UK, the Royal College of Speech and Language Therapists (RCSLT) guidelines advise that before voice therapy is undertaken by an SLT, the patient should be examined by their GP and should undergo endoscopic evaluation of the larynx by an Otolaryngologist or highly specialised clinician, either as a separate procedure or as part of a multidisciplinary voice clinic. This evaluation should take place less than six months prior to initial speech and language therapy contact. The clinician is then aware of the results of this examination, with regard to the vocal fold appearance, a description of the free edge of the vocal folds, the approximation on phon-ation and mobility characteristics.

Services should ensure good availability of multidisciplinary joint voice clinic services, which provide an invaluable resource in the identification and management of voice disorders. Multidisciplinary voice clinics can help improve the accuracy of voice-related diagnoses, reduce the risk of inappropriate interventions and in terms of service delivery and commissioning are cost-effective (Phillips *et al.*, 2005; British Voice Association, 2012). Given the developments in healthcare provision and the extended role of the therapy prac-titioner, some clinics already accept referrals directly to the speech and language therapy specialist. The SLT-led clinic for Endoscopic Evaluation of the Larynx will be discussed in Chapter 8.

Hearing acuity

Hearing may be a relevant contributing factor to dysphonia, where the patient has reduced self-monitoring of pitch, volume and quality of voice and may use excess effort with increased volume to ensure being heard. Conversely, some hearing-impaired patients produce quiet, inadequate voice with little output of airflow in voice production, thus producing an aero-dynamic disturbance and dysphonia. In other instances, profoundly deaf adults have been known to use raised pitch, resulting in fatigue, weakness and loss of tone in the vocal fold musculature. Similarly, the increased anxiety and tension, which may be caused by failure of others to understand the communication of the hearing-impaired adult, can result in a MTD. It is imperative, therefore, if there is any question of hearing disturbance, that a full assessment is made by the audiologist. Consideration should also be given to the potential presence of presbycusis (gradual hearing loss) in an older patient as a common feature of ageing. About 30–35% of adults age 65 and older have a hearing loss and it is estimated that 40–50% of people aged 75 and older have a hearing loss.

Because the process of loss of hearing is gradual, people who have presbycusis may not realise that their hearing is diminishing and as sounds become less and less clear and lower in volume those patients experiencing this themselves, or in a partner, may begin to use increased vocal volume with accompanied vocal tension.

Vocal health

Optimal voice use, whether for speech or singing, requires a healthy and mobile vocal tract, with sufficient stamina and flexibility for the patient's daily voice tasks. It is therefore essential to identify any intermittent, chronic or acute factors that may compromise the health of the mucosal linings and be manifest as irritation, increased secretions, throat clearing, gastro-oesophageal reflux disorder (GORD) or laryngopharyngeal reflux (LPR). Patients may report episodes of no voice disturbance but of discomfort, dryness, irritation, dry cough, throat clearing, a feeling of a 'lump in the throat', difficulty swallowing or neck discomfort. Lenderking *et al.* (2003) described many of these symptoms as being those commonly associated with LPR.

Questions regarding vocal health should also explore the frequency and severity of the symptom plus any common factors noted when symptoms occur, so that a picture is gradually compiled of the circumstances and timescales most frequently associated with discomfort or disorder in the health of the vocal tract. The patient's description of the vocal tract and its health will then contribute to and facilitate appropriate management of the presenting symptoms, aiming to reduce contributing and perpetuating factors in the voice disorder.

Vocal care

Care of the voice is unfortunately not commonly acknowledged as important by many people, even those who use voice professionally or occupationally, with many completely unaware of the vocal behaviours which lead to vocal misuse and which are part of their lifestyle. It is therefore vital to collate information on awareness of vocal care and issues that may affect or compromise voice production, such as shouting, smoking, alcohol or caffeine intake, hydration and dietary habits. As already noted, the clinician should support the patient as far as is possible towards smoking cessation and reduction in alcohol intake with preventative health leaflets and advice. This section is very closely related to Vocal Health with various aspects from each topic being interrelated; for example, eating spicy food resulting in a dry mouth and thirst or eating foods with thick, creamy sauces or a high carbohydrate content leading to thick secretions and increased throat clearing. While the importance of hydration is now more generally recognised, many patients may still remain unaware of the detrimental effect of systematic dehydration on voice production (Martin and Darnley, 2019). It is, unfortunately, still not uncommon to find patients who drink little or no water, including that in tea, coffee or cordials on a daily basis. It may not be known that high caffeine intake should also be avoided, as it is a diuretic and can also result in dehydration with consequent irritation to the vocal folds. Older patients may resist drinking enough fluid because of bladder control or issues such as stress, urge, or functionary urinary incontinence. It is important for the clinician to gently explore this issue if dehydration is considered a key factor in the maintenance of the voice disorder. Appendix I provides a number of voice care recommendations as a guide for patients.

Vocal demand

The relationship between heavy vocal demand and potential vocal misuse has been recognised for many years, especially in occupations where vocal demand is high as in teaching, telesales, health and leisure industries (Fontan *et al.*, 2016). Many of these occupations are vocally intensive, necessitating frequent and prolonged periods of loud phonation without sufficient recovery time. Titze (2001) suggests the following critical risk factors associated with excessive vocalisation: duration of exposure, frequency of vibration and vocal loudness.

It is, however, important to note the paradox that despite heavy vocal demands some individuals are able to sustain phonation without compromising quality. Cooper's view (1973) that 'Voice Disorders are not due to overuse of the voice; they are due to misuse and abuse of the voice. A voice well used is essentially never overused' remains equally valid today as it was almost half a century ago.

Vocal status

A patient's perception of his/her voice may vary considerably, especially with regard to how voice has altered and the parameters in which it has altered. Similarly, there can be common misunderstandings of words such as 'loudness' and 'pitch'; for example, the question 'Is your voice lower now?' may convey either pitch or intensity to different people. It is therefore helpful to use questions to encourage the patient regarding perception of voice change, voice quality, stamina and flexibility of voice. This will, of course, be supplemented by the clinician's perceptual assessment and instrumentation. Where terminology is unfamiliar to patients, the clinician may need to be creative in describing, for example, voice or pitch breaks as sudden changes in voice to higher or lower pitch, to a whisper and back to voice again, or even demonstrating the nature of the voice or pitch break. It can be difficult to understand the impact of experiencing a quality of voice which is out of one's control, which is harsh, hoarse, rough, breathy or whispery. The daily use of voice can be an unhappy experience for some patients when it involves a changed voice quality which is perceived as unpleasant and 'not my voice', with the implication that the voice does not convey the 'real' person or indeed does not 'belong' to the patient.

Voice geneogram

Part of the whole picture of the patient and their voice involves those influences which may affect or compromise voice use, such as family and cultural values, and social training, as these determine an individual's view of themselves and how they relate to those around them. The voice serves to reflect not only the patient's emotional state and personality, but also their physical state and previous life history and experience.

For most patients, voice is a valued and central part of their identity. It is therefore important not only to look at a patient's current lifestyle and personality, but also to examine what previous experiences have shaped his/her world view, view of him/herself and communicative competence. Even small changes in the manner or production of speech will have an effect on vocal quality, so before promoting change in vocal quality it is important to assess a patient's ability to recognise and monitor voice quality and vocal habits. For example, how much does the patient value and identify with his/her own voice? How well can the patient perceive and monitor both his/her and others' vocal quality? How much, if at all, were there imposed changes in the patient's speech patterns with consequent change in vocal quality?

Anxiety and stress

The relationship between voice, emotion and physical state has been well documented. Authors such as Morrison and Rammage (2000), Andrews (2006) and Colton *et al.* (2011) reference factors such as personality characteristics, emotional reactions to acute or chronic life stressors and emotional disturbances, such as chronic anxiety. These affect the movement of the vocal folds through increased levels of intrinsic and extrinsic laryngeal muscle tension.

In any discussion of stress with the patient, it is important to try to define what is understood by the term 'stress'. To introduce this subject, it may be helpful to outline the relationship between stress and muscular tension, the impact of stress on various physical systems and specific impact on phonation and voice quality. It is then less threatening to ask the patient the simple question, 'Have you had particular areas of stress in the past year – you need not tell me the details, just if it has occurred?' Initially patients will often answer the latter part of the question, but then continue to expand on the detail of their response.

Returning to the wisdom of Aronson (1990b), I am grateful to Annie Elias for this quote:

> If we do not ask, and the patient does not volunteer the information, which they almost never do, then what other conclusion can we draw than that they have no psychologically related voice disorder? Our thinking becomes circular. If we do not ask about psychological problems, we do not hear about them. If we do not hear about them, we do not believe in them. And, if we do not believe in them, we do not ask about them.

Many people have never been encouraged to share at a deep level or describe emotional issues, although it is encouraging to note that this situation is changing and issues of mental health are much less stigmatised than was previously the case. Patients may have real difficulties in knowing how to properly express their inner emotion in words and the whole story may take some time to unfold. It is important that the patient feels an acceptance of what is being shared and of their reaction to life's circumstances. Often patients will say, 'I should not feel this way' and need to be reassured that the expression of emotion is acceptable. Clinicians must remember that for many people discussing personal issues, or even expressing opinions and emotions about personal situations, is an entirely new experience in their life. Neither must it be assumed that because there is difficulty in accessing the information, the patient is withholding something. Questions must not become an interrogation but should be sensitive in unravelling the complexities of relationships and unearthing the relevance of the story. As the practical information is pieced together, it becomes easier to interject questions such as, 'How do you feel about that?' or 'Are you concerned about that?' to unearth possible stress factors and to get to know the patient. At a later stage, if stress proves to be a major contributing factor, it may be helpful to explore the various reactions and responses of the patient to different stimuli or different events. By doing so, the clinician aims to assist self-awareness in patients, so enabling them to establish strategies for therapeutic change. In some instances, however, there may well be a need for further referral to an appropriate agency, but a decision on this will more easily be made if the clinician and patient have arrived at it together.

Social functioning

Once the patient has been able to find a way in which to share this quite personal information with the clinician, the clinician can then move on to address the patient's leisure activities and social contacts through gentle open questions such as, 'Can you tell me something about your leisure activities?', 'When you think about your social life how would you describe it?', 'Thinking about your friends, can you tell me a little about where you would usually meet up with them?'

The frequency and type of leisure activities may provide further information on vocal loading in sports, vocal effort in a particular movement during a sport, posture during an activity and the amount of physical demand involved. Social contacts are often in a noisy and sometimes smoky environment and may also regularly involve a group with several simultaneous discussions taking place. Details of the surrounding environment, background music and participation of the audience may all provide valuable information to contributing factors in the voice disorder. While the incidence of recreational drug use is increasing, clinicians should use their own judgement on the appropriate questions to pose. It may be unwise in some situations to raise the issue of drug use, while in others it would be quite an acceptable subject. Anything which may have an impact on health is vital information in the case-history compilation and should be addressed at some point in the therapy process.

Not only should the clinician access information on the patient's voice use during social and leisure activities but they must explore any effect of the voice disorder on the patient's usual social involvement because patients may withdraw from their habitual contacts. Some patients may become frustrated if they feel that they are repeatedly being asked if they have a cold or if their throat is sore. Similarly, it can become simply too much effort to participate socially if the patient cannot be heard over background noise, leading to frustration and potentially increased voice misuse. As already noted in Chapter 1, social isolation is a source of distress, reduced communication opportunities and limitations in important quality-of-life domains.

Employment and work environment

For those in work this can provide critical clues to contributing factors. The subject might be introduced by asking questions such as: 'And your work. Tell me about that and what it involves.' In addition to the questions in the VIP, an Occupational Environmental and Acoustic Checklist is provided in Appendix II for patients to complete to highlight some of the challenges they may encounter in their occupational roles which, it is hoped, will better inform the clinician and provide opportunities for change. It is also hoped that in bringing together a number of factors that affect voice related to the employment and work environment, it will provide insight for the patient as to the multiple factors that may have contributed to and maintained their voice disorder.

Acoustics and noise levels

The clinician hopes to have a clear picture of the patient's working situation, with an understanding of the physical challenges to communication in the layout and acoustics of, for example, the factory, office or classroom. Some patients may work in a variety of spaces throughout the day, with the demand for compensatory vocal techniques for the different acoustics within each space. Similarly, the structure of buildings and the materials used inside them will determine the acoustic properties of the space. In general, low ceilings, carpeted floors, covered walls and soft furnishings tend to 'dampen and deaden' sound and consequently absorb the voice. Hard surfaces such as varnished timber or wooden tiles, steel-framed windows and doors, large expanses of glass and bare walls tend to produce a bright, sharp and occasionally echoing sound. A good acoustic environment provides conditions in which noise is suppressed and speech is clear and words are easily distinguishable (Martin and Darnley, 2019). For patients who fall into the occupational voice user (OVU) status (Chapter 2) it is important to carefully question them about the acoustic environment in which they work and if necessary recommend that if there are acoustic problems in the work setting that they look to bring in acoustic professionals to help alleviate some of the acoustic difficulties. In the same way that ergonomic or health and safety issues would be dealt with by an employer, so too acoustic difficulties should be examined as they have an impact on the vocal health of the patient.

Use of protective equipment and amplification

The habitual noise level, even when within health and safety guidelines, may result in demands on voice or hearing if the patient has inadequate voice projection. Equally, some employers may adhere to all health and safety conditions, only to find that their employees fail to utilise ear protection or masks because they find them uncomfortable. Fontan *et al.* (2016) reported on a study of self-reported vocal difficulties in sports and fitness instructors (SFIs). The results indicated a prevalence of 55% and the Voice Handicap Index was significantly associated with gender, age and variables related to work environment (noise and music) and habits (shouting, frequency of classes), as well as with daily sleeping time. Results also indicate that a minority of the SFIs (37%) received information on vocal difficulties, whereas a majority (80%) declared being interested in participating in prevention programmes. This work identified SFI as a high-risk population for voice disorders and supports the results of Long *et al.* (1998), who almost 20 years earlier found that 44% of aerobics instructors had partial or complete voice loss during and after instructing.

Background noise, which may be within or external to the immediate environment, may result in high-level vocal demand. Also, vocal loading in some domestic or care situations may be even higher than in many work circumstances and questions relating to voice use must be perceptive.

Ventilation, heating and pollution

The effect of dryness of the upper respiratory tract is commonly experienced, resulting in irritation and frequent coughing. Working in an environment which has poor ventilation or poor temperature control may lead to a chronic dryness in the tract and particularly in the vocal folds. Similarly, the effects of dust, pollution, fumes, smoke and industrial materials must also be considered. Most patients are very aware of the conditions in their immediate situation and can describe the extent of their control over this. As with other aspects of vocal 'health and safety', it is important to closely question patients regarding this aspect of their working environment.

Hours and conditions of work, the length and number of breaks

What may seem a good working situation for a few hours of the day may become intolerable over many hours, with a limited number of breaks from the immediate environment. This, of course, may be just as relevant in the home with a demanding care situation as it is in any work environment. The clinician may need to ask various searching and specific questions to discover the detail, because what is familiar and accepted as the 'norm' may not be deemed by the patient as having any relevance.

Postural demands

The effect on posture is still overlooked by some employers and employees despite the dissemination of ergonomic information. Static posture for lengthy periods of time can be commonplace in many occupations. In addition to the ergonomic challenges on the voice of the workplace in terms of seating and work station furniture, so too is the extensive use of tablets, laptops and phones not only for work but also for personal use. Data for mobile phone use in 2019 suggests that individuals spend on average 3 hours and 15 minutes per day on their phones (Matei, 2019). Such significant periods of time spent looking down at smart phones or tablets inevitably compromises head/neck alignment. Apart from the generalised stiffness and discomfort experienced, there is also the impact on the voice as alterations in the head–neck–spine relationship occurs and changes to the position of the larynx within the pharynx results. Vocal quality is thus compromised, leading to a rather squeezed sound. The impact of inappropriate or incorrect posture should therefore be considered very carefully by the clinician as a potential contributing factor.

Summary

It has been mentioned previously that the author's preference is to use the Voice Impact Profile because much of the above information can be gained through its use and can be supplemented at subsequent sessions as more information is unearthed. If conventional case-history taking is employed, it may well be difficult to gather all the above information in one session and the full picture will build over a period of time.

However, whatever method of interviewing and case-history taking is involved, the clinician must find his/her own style. With experience and practice, the style evolves and is natural, the patient is at ease and communicates at the optimal level.

ASSESSMENT

Introduction

Voice assessment procedures will differ from country to country and different weighting may well be given to certain aspects of the assessment depending on the healthcare system within which clinicians practice. In the UK, for example, the RCSLT lays down strict criteria for the initial assessment phase – such as the principles underpinning assessment; standards and guidance around the initial assessment stage; timing of the assessment; involvement of others in the assessment and the form of the assessment – while the Health and Care Professions Council (HCPC) supervises standards of proficiency of those clinicians who are registered with them. So too, the American Speech Language Hearing Association (ASHA) has a protocol on assessment tools, techniques and data sources. In other countries assessment protocols and information will be available for their members to follow.

Perceptual assessment

Best practice would encourage a comprehensive assessment, consistent with the World Health Organization's (WHO) International Classification of Functioning, Disability and Health (ICF) framework (WHO, 2001). The assessment should use both standardised and non-standardised measures and contain a mix of subjective and objective perceptual and acoustic measurements to be used by the clinician as part of the diagnostic process to augment information from other sources, such as the case history. The basic universal principle underpinning assessment is that assessment is informed by the best available evidence and authorised by patient consent. It is, of course critical that, as was noted in Chapter 4, all aspects of the assessment process fulfil the requirements of information documentation, such as gaining the patient's permission to make acoustic and visual recordings of the session, secure storage of the data and to what use they may be put. This may differ from clinic to clinic, but it is imperative that clinicians are aware of procedures. It is important to see assessment as part of an ongoing process, which does not remain separate to, but is part of, intervention. As the ongoing clinician/patient partnership develops, further information gathering or self-disclosure by the patient influence the clinician's thinking. This informs the diagnostic process and leads to adaptation of the intervention pathway. Of critical importance is to continue to 'take the patient with you' as you continue along the assessment process that began with building the patient profile, the topic of Chapter 4. The importance of reflecting the patient's own assessment of how the voice problem affects their emotions and self image and their ability to communicate effectively in everyday activities is of paramount importance and should be at the forefront of any perceptual assessment.

A *Voice Assessment Sheet* is contained in Appendix VI which identifies areas that will ensure the clinician can build a comprehensive picture of the patient's current vocal competencies at the time of assessment. This is a subjective auditory–perceptual assessment of voice quality, based on clinical impressions by the clinician, which looks at specific areas of voice quality in detail. It should be emphasised that any assessment procedure should be explained in as clear and concise a manner as possible. As with any new task, it is important to ensure not only that patients understand completely what they are being asked to do, but also that the task is designed in manageable sections. If a patient does not manage to understand essential elements of the task or cannot participate, a different explanation should be given or a different task design should be instigated. Another aspect which is sometimes overlooked is the patient's desire to 'do well' and their accompanying anxiety can create undue tension. If this occurs, the patient's true ability may be disguised and it will be difficult to discriminate between the successful completion of the task, representing true ability, and a task 'performance'. At all times it is important for the clinician to note, in keeping with the WHO ICF framework, any impairment in body structure and function, comorbid deficits, limitations in activity and participation, contextual factors and quality of life issues.

During the assessment it is very important that the clinician maintains visual contact with the patient so that any non-verbal behaviour associated with the voice disorder is noted. The non-verbal behaviour may range, for example, from facial grimacing which indicates pain, breath holding, lack of ability to maintain eye contact, subtle indications of articulatory groping or facial tension. Some of these signals of pain or discomfort will be fleeting and subtle, others will be more overt. The extent of the response may not necessarily equate with the discomfort experienced. Often individuals mask discomfort most successfully, particularly if it is long-standing, while others may have become habituated to the discomfort. It is usually recommended that note-taking be kept to a minimum, so that any diagnostic clues can be observed. For less-experienced clinicians, note-taking is perfectly acceptable, providing it is fairly discreet and does not interfere with the flow of the assessment.

Colton *et al.* (2011) suggest that patients with voice problems tend to present with nine major symptoms, cited below.

- *Hoarseness*: reflecting aperiodicity of vocal fold vibration. Some patients will use the word 'hoarse' to refer to this symptom, some will use terms such as 'rough' or 'raspy' voice.

- *Vocal fatigue*: patients state that they feel tired after prolonged talking and often say that continued talking requires a great deal of effort.
- *Breathy voice*: patients report that they are unable to complete sentences without running out of air and additionally that they have difficulty in being heard, especially in noisy situations.
- *Reduced phonational range*: patients report that they experience difficulty producing notes that were previously no problem. This symptom is usually associated with singers.
- *Aphonia*: patients speak in a whisper and complain of effortful voicing.
- *Pitch breaks or inappropriately high pitch*: patients may complain of periodic 'squeakiness' or of voice 'cracks'. They do not know what sound will come out.
- *Strain/struggle voice*: these patients report that it is difficult to talk and additionally may be unable to initiate or maintain voice. They experience a great deal of tension when speaking and become tired due to the effort involved.
- *Tremor*: patients report that the voice is 'wobbly' or 'shaky' and they are unable to voluntarily produce a sustained sound. The 'shaky' voice is usually consistent in its disturbance.
- *Pain and other physical sensations*: there are varying reports about pain, some patients localising the pain, others reporting more generalised pain. Patients will also often report vague feelings of discomfort and a feeling of dryness, heat and irritation in the area of the larynx.

Many of these symptoms will be apparent as the assessment process (below) unfolds, either singly or, more likely, as reflected by Colton *et al.* (2011), in combination.

The assessment process

Posture

Posture is of critical importance in maximising vocal potential and it is an area that should be carefully assessed. Symmetry and asymmetry are useful watch words as these descriptors of posture can offer a useful shorthand for the clinician and at the same time alert the clinician to aspects of the patient's vocal quality. It is important to look at posture in both sitting and standing positions. Is the patient's posture over-corrected, over-erect or slumped with shoulders hunched and head thrust forward? It is important to note aspects such as eye levels, head/neck alignment, the angle at which the head is carried. Is there evident asymmetry in any aspect of the patient's physicality which could affect voice to some degree? Of course, as part of assessing a patient's posture the clinician should also be aware of the mind–body–voice connection. As well as the physiological impact on voice quality, posture can give many clues about the individual's emotional state and how they value themselves. A confident and open posture will generally be perceived as positive, whereas a slumped or stooped posture with lowered eye levels (in the absence of a physical infirmity or illness) is usually judged negatively. These judgements, which may be seen as 'value' judgements, nevertheless often give a silent but powerful indication as to the true emotional state of the patient.

When assessing 'performers', from occupational voice user to the elite singer, such as an opera singer, or the elite voice user such as an actor, it is particularly important to assess their 'performance' posture carefully. They may have unconsciously adopted a posture which imposes stress or strain on the laryngeal musculature. Chapman (2017) suggests that when a singer walks onstage, especially onto the concert platform, their posture gives an immediate and subtle message to the audience and from this message the audience has a certain expectation. A visual record can be particularly helpful in identifying specific performance habits such as turning the head slightly to a fixed microphone or compensatory movements of the head and neck which may become habitual when using hand-held microphones. Multimedia is now so ubiquitous that YouTube, for example, will inevitably throw up past recordings of performers in action and it is particularly helpful for monitoring postural change over a period of months or years. Some of these changes may be unconscious but may be the result of compensatory movements as a consequence of pain, discomfort or fatigue. Assessment of posture is important in all performance media, from solo concert performance to musical theatre, and any assessment should consider wide-ranging aspects such as the extent of movement while vocalising, staging, space restriction and costume. This is important both in musical theatre, where actors are required to sing, move and perform at the same time, and in opera where singers increasingly need to act and move vigorously around the stage. The professional voice user also needs to be aware of the demands of the space in which they are performing. Some performance staging requires the actor or singer to work in a small space or in a physically challenging position. Sometimes actors and singers work on a raked stage which requires a conscious postural readjustment in order not to throw the vocal tract out of alignment. Similarly, heavy, constricting costumes, corsets, wigs and shoes often present vocal challenges as they are rarely designed to take vocal demands into account, unlike in ballet where costumes are specifically designed not to compromise performance in any way. Chapman (2017) reminds the reader of the need to target abdominal muscles not only for postural alignment and core stability but also for their role in the management and support of breath for singing.

Breathing/respiratory pattern

For many patients, shallow breathing patterns are a feature of their voice disorder, causing problems of vocal support, restricting the aerodynamic contribution to vocal fold vibration and creating problems of prosody. In the author's opinion, breathing remains critical in terms of supporting the voice and needs to be assessed and modified, although this is a view that is not shared by all clinicians. Colton *et al.* (2011), for example, suggest that a great deal more emphasis has been placed on teaching or correcting breathing than is usually necessary unless the patient is a professional voice user. The author would agree that in some instances too much focus on the teaching of breathing may set up sites of tension, but at the same time argues that it is an important entry into aspects such as release of tension, achieving the synchrony of breathing and voicing, and allows for attention to the patient's economic use of breath. The clinician will learn much from observation, watching the patient while taking a case history or in general pre-assessment conversation with the patient. The clinician should note whether the patient at rest tends to use the nose or mouth for breathing. It is also important to look at breathing rate, noting whether this is steady and regular. In addition, any breathlessness or respiratory stridor should be noted and if present then additional care must be taken with any breathing assessment. Ask the individual to gradually slow and deepen breathing, preferably when standing, and watch for movement in the shoulders, neck, upper chest and abdomen. How does the individual take in the breath? Is this a gasping, constricted intake or a slower, more normal in-breath?

The respiratory patterns most usually identified are as follows.

Clavicular or upper chest breathing, where the patient raises the shoulders, elevates the clavicles with concomitant movement in the neck muscles. Indeed, the muscles may often 'stand out' with the effort involved. Many patients will also raise the ribcage, resulting in increased muscle tension. This method allows for very minimal intake and reduced vocal support. Clavicular breathing may be noted when patients are tense and anxious and may be ill-prepared for the assessment process. It is for that reason that the instruction to the patient should be, as noted above, 'gradually slow and deepen your breath' rather than simply ask them to 'take in a deep breath'. While there may be limited robust data to support the view that clavicular breathing is a symptom or sign of voice problems, clinicians should be aware that clavicular breathing may be a symptom of asthma, chronic obstructive pulmonary disease (COPD), a neurological disorder or in fact tension and anxiety.

Thoracic breathing, where the patient expands the mid-thoracic area during inspiration, resulting in little expansion of the lower thoracic and abdominal cavities. The lack of abdominal movement will be clearly noted. This is the most frequently used method of breathing generally used for quiet, at-rest breathing or breathing for life. This method does not, however, allow sufficient expansion of the lungs for heavy vocal demands as the thoracic cage limits lung mobility.

Diaphragmatic breathing, where the patient expands the abdominal muscles to allow for a downward displacement of the diaphragm, is combined with the expansion of the lungs by outward movement of the lower ribs. There is little movement of the shoulders. This method allows for the greatest expansion of the lungs with a consequent increase in the volume of air inhaled. Professional voice users will often have learned this method of breathing (see above; Chapman, 2017), but it is a less usual method for inexperienced voice users.

Degree of general body tension

This is, to some extent, the most subjective measurement and relies very much on the visual impression gained by the clinician when taking the case history and the ensuing discussion. Consideration should be given to posture. Is the patient sitting on the edge of the chair? Are they grasping the arms of the chair? Are the hands clasped tightly together? Do they move constantly? Are the shoulders habitually raised or is there a constant change of position? In addition, note the patient's facial expression. Is there limited facial expression? Are there any involuntary facial tics? The latter can, of course, relate to an underlying neurological condition but extreme tension and/or anxiety may also evince these symptoms.

Tongue, jaw and neck tension

Tension in the tongue and jaw is often an accompanying feature of general body tension, particularly neck tension. In some patients the neck and supralaryngeal strap muscles stand out as the patient speaks. Tension is, of course, very difficult to measure and there is little available objective data to determine what is unacceptable in terms of normal voicing, although it is usual for voice production to be fairly effortless. What is important, however, is that the clinician notes any undue tension and reflects on potential causes; is this tension related to hyperfunctional voice use, or might it be a compensatory behaviour with its roots in a neurological disorder or laryngeal pathology?

Undue tension in the jaw muscles will affect articulation and resonance, while little or no mandibular movement creates problems in the manner and place of articulation, as the tongue has to play an increased compensatory role. Tension in the tongue, especially if it is retracted, may occlude the pharynx and, as a result, resonance will be affected with a resultant hollow-sounding or cul-de-sac resonance heard. In contrast, if the tongue is carried too far forward, the voice lacks the resonance of the back vowels. In order to assess tension in the mandible, restricted jaw movement and lack of jaw opening should be observed. This can be felt by placing fingers on either side of the face, level with the temporo-mandibular joint. Tension in the root of the tongue may be felt by pressing gently under the chin and assessing plasticity. In addition, the patient may be asked to phonate /ah/ and see if the tongue is retracted. Is the patient aware of jaw clenching or teeth grinding?

Laryngeal and pharyngeal tension

Various assessment methods, clinical, radiological and electromyography, have been used to measure laryngeal muscular tension in patients. The commonly used methods for evaluation and diagnosis are, however, clinical, which includes case history, observational techniques and palpation. If the neck area is palpated, information regarding the status of the extrinsic laryngeal musculature and the positions of the major laryngeal cartilages at rest may be gained (Mathieson *et al.*, 2009). A more detailed description and efficacy of perilaryngeal manual therapy is included in Chapter 7. If patients report laryngeal pain in the absence of any vocal pathology it is important to establish the site of the pain and to examine potential indicators of laryngeal tension, such as elevation of the hyoid bone and elevation of the larynx. Deem and Miller (2000) suggest that the degree of laryngeal tension is directly proportional to (a) the amount of elevation of the laryngeal structures and (b) the amount of pain reported by the patient. The Vocal Tract Discomfort Scale (VTDS; Mathieson *et al.*, 2007) is a very useful tool as part of patient profiling, as it allows the patient to identify the symptoms they are experiencing in the throat and to narrow down the frequency and severity of the symptoms/sensations using a numerical scale. It is also important to establish if the patient tends to maintain a high tongue forward position even when the tongue is at rest. Evidence of laryngeal tension may also be noted in a strained or pressed vocal quality with periods of vocal or hard attack.

Vocal or hard attack

Phonation which starts abruptly with hard glottal attack can be identified quite easily and assessed on a present/absent basis. Hard glottal attack is particularly noticeable on vowels. Ask the patient to say a sentence with several vowels, for example, 'Any apples for Andrew?' and listen for any abrupt adduction of the vocal folds. Laryngeal compression and pharyngeal constriction may also be a feature of hard glottal attack and it is important to note either of these features.

Vocal support

Asking the patient to take a breath and sustain the production of /s/ for as long as possible gives an indication of how much air support they have for voice and how efficiently the individual can control expiration. Record the time in seconds. As a guide, one might expect an adult to sustain /s/ for approximately 20 seconds, but it is most unlikely that many voice patients will achieve this time. It is, however, important to recognise that within this task certain additional features need to be assessed. For example, a patient could produce a very low volume /s/ for 15 seconds, but this would not necessarily translate into vocal efficiency in response to vocal demands in continuous speech or when attempting to use the voice at high volume. It is also important to listen when the patient is speaking. Are they squeezing out a small amount of air without replenishing the supply? An inadequate airflow may be indicative of a problem and should be investigated.

Phonation time

Maximum phonation time (MPT) refers to the maximum time an individual can sustain a sound on one breath following a maximum inspiration. The patient is asked to take a breath and then sustain the production of /z/ for as long as possible. Again, note the time in seconds. As with the vocal support time, one would, as a guide, expect an adult male to sustain the sound for approximately 25–35 seconds and an adult female for 15–25 seconds (Speyer *et al.*, 2010). It should be noted that it is rare for most voice patients to be able to sustain phonation for this length of time. It is also important to note that some patients may require several 'trials' at this task as this assessment is quite alien to most people, so it is important to model the task to patients in advance and give clear instructions to the patient. A study by Maslan *et al.* (2011) reported that in a cohort of older adults many could phonate for at least 20 seconds in the absence of pathology and supported the findings of Bless and Hirano (1982) that three trials were usually sufficient for accurate MPT measures. Patients with no respiratory problems and no vocal fold pathology are usually able to sustain /s/ and /z/ for the same length of time, achieving a ratio of one, but in cases of vocal fold pathology the s/z ratio is sharply increased (Boone and McFarlane, 1988) as the discrepancy between sustained voiceless and voiced sounds (s and z) becomes greater. An s/z ratio greater than 1:4 may, they suggest, indicate a vocal pathology. During the assessment, the clinician should note additionally any periods of devoicing, intermittent voicing and sustained voicing during spontaneous speech.

Production of reflexive sounds

Assessment of reflexive/vegetative sounds, which include laughing, coughing, clearing the throat and fillers such as /em/ or /uh-huh/ are important indicators of voice quality produced in a non-speech task. This assessment can give the clinician useful information, as many patients do not perceive the production of reflexive sounds as using the voice. It is important to compare how and if the quality, pitch and loudness of the voice differs from that which the patient produces on speech tasks. It is also useful to assess the amount of energy the patient utilises for these tasks, particularly on throat clearing. It is likely that patients will have already spontaneously produced some reflexive sounds and these should have been noted by the clinician and can be a useful comparison with those produced on demand.

Pitch/voice placement

In this section the clinician should look at four different but interacting aspects of pitch: habitual pitch, pitch range, pitch breaks and pitch variation.

Habitual pitch

Habitual pitch (modal frequency range) refers to the pitch that is most used by the patient in everyday speech. This can be measured by a speech sample recorded during conversation or the use of a standard passage such as 'The Rainbow Passage' (Fairbanks, 1960). It is also important to refer to patients for feedback on pitch changes they have noted or that friends, colleagues or family have reported back to them. Low pitch does not mean a disorder; longitudinal change is the most important criterion.

Pitch range

The patient's vocal range should be assessed. It is important to note whether the range is restricted or whether the patient can produce notes at both ends of their range. Often notes at the high end of the range are difficult for patients to achieve and these may be reported anecdotally as having been 'lost'. It is much rarer for patients to 'lose' notes at the lower end of their scale. It is, however, important to recognise that while many professional singers will report that their full range is not restricted, further questioning will reveal that the quality of certain pitches has been altered. Within this section it is also important to assess whether the pitch range is appropriate to the age and sex of the patient. It should also be remembered that variations occur due to ethnic and cultural mores in terms of pitch, so clinicians should be alert to the fact that a perceptual judgement of pitch can be affected by aspects other than voice quality characteristics. The vexed question of optimum pitch, in other words 'the frequency of vocal fold movement that allows optimal resonance with least vocal effort', should perhaps be addressed here. Many clinicians do not believe in the concept of optimum pitch. Colton *et al.* (2011) call it 'the myth of optimum pitch', but there does seem to be adequate clinical evidence that there are certain points in the pitch range where a patient will suggest that their voice 'feels comfortable' and 'sounds best' (Deem and Miller, 2000). It must, however, be remembered that any change in quality is a factor of both the sound source and the resonating cavity, so it is important not to reinforce either inappropriate pitch or distortion in the resonating cavities simply because the voice 'sounds better'.

Pitch breaks

Unexpected or uncontrolled upward or downward shifts in pitch are often associated with the adolescent male voice, but they are also symptomatic of laryngeal pathologies or changes at the level of neural control of phonation, for example, in Parkinson's disease, multiple sclerosis or motor neurone disease. These pitch breaks can be readily perceived by even the most inexperienced listener.

Pitch variation

A lack of pitch variation can be a symptom of neurological impairment or it can be an indication of depression or psychosis. It is, however, important as a diagnostic indicator to differentiate between the individual who can vary pitch and does not do so, and the individual who is actually unable to do so.

Voice projection

This is an assessment of how appropriately patients project their voice and regulate volume. A reduction in volume may also be symptomatic of a tight, held-back breathing method so it is important to identify the cause correctly. Although loudness variations may be the result of impairment, they may also be the result of habit, personality or family dynamics. For some patients, particularly those with hyperfunction, excessive volume is only one feature of their total problem. At the other extreme, some patients will become too quiet as a result of, for example, deafness where, due to their inability to monitor loudness levels and in order not to 'shout', they may become inappropriately quiet with little or no projection. For some individuals a lack of volume is a symptom of an underlying pathology, for example, vocal fold paralysis, or may be indicative of neurological impairment such as Parkinson's disease or bulbar palsy, where the voice will be soft and barely audible. The clinician should assess on a perceptual scale of 'too loud to too soft', bearing in mind that a judgement on loudness levels is speaking-situation-dependent and may not reflect habitual loudness levels.

Articulatory precision

Articulatory precision should be considered within a voice assessment battery as it offers important diagnostic information regarding what Mathieson (2001) refers to as 'organic and behavioural elements' of voice disorders. Articulatory precision, or lack of it, will add important detail to the assessment process with regard to the patient's ability to judge, monitor and produce an appropriate degree of muscular effort needed to initiate specific movement of the articulators. Both excessive and/or limited muscular effort should be recognised and evaluated. For example, excessive muscular effort in the articulators may be indicated by overly precise lip movement or bunching of the tongue during speech, while lack of precision, sluggish movement, difficulty in sustaining lip seal or hyponasal resonance may indicate difficulty in recruiting sufficient muscle tone, strength or speed. Neurological disease such as Parkinson's disease, multiple sclerosis, motor neurone disease or myasthenia gravis may initially manifest as a disordered vocal quality or articulatory imprecision and for that reason it is essential that the clinician includes potential central nervous system lesions in any differential diagnostic assessment.

Severity rating

GRBAS (Hirano, 1981), an acronym for Grade, Roughness, Breathy, Aesthenic, Strained, is a rating scale which has found mainstream recognition as a reliable measure and is now accepted as a universal rating standard. Other perceptual ratings of voice quality such as Consensus Auditory Perceptual Evaluation of Voice (CAPE-V; Kempster *et al.*, 2009) are, of course, available. Severity rating is intimately connected to vocal handicap issues, of which several assessments are available to clinicians (e.g. Jacobson *et al.*, 1997; Hogikyan and Sethuraman, 1999; Ma and Yiu, 2001)

The patient's perception of the severity of the voice disorder may be very different from the clinician's perception of the disorder. As Ma and Yiu (2001) noted, 'the self-perceived voice problem had little correlation with the degree of voice-quality impairment measured acoustically and perceptually by speech pathologists'. Not only is it important to note this but also to see the significance of this apparent 'perceptual gulf' with respect to differential diagnosis. Clinicians may identify as 'quite severe' a voice disorder about which a patient may show little or no concern. The *Voice Disability Coping Questionnaire* (VDCQ; Epstein *et al.*, 2009) is a tool for assessing specific coping strategies used by patients with dysphonia. The opening question in the *Voice Skills Perceptual Profile* (Shewell, 2009) is: 'Can you describe the sound and feeling of your voice, and why you are here?' The *Vocal Tract Discomfort Scale* (VTD; Mathieson *et al.*, 2009) was developed as a tool to quantify the severity and frequency of a patient's throat discomfort using qualitative descriptors. It is a patient self-rating scale completed before palpatory evaluation (see laryngeal and pharyngeal tension above).

Patient-reported outcome (PRO) measures, defined as 'any report of the status of a patient's health condition that comes directly from the patient without interpretation of the patient's response by a clinician or anyone else' (Reeve *et al.*, 2013; Snyder *et al.*, 2013), provide a method of systematically capturing patient perspective and experience. PRO measures are increasingly used to better understand the perspectives of, and to measure concepts that matter to, the patient (Patrick *et al.*, 2007). The ICFDH paradigm (WHO, 2001) is considered the international standard for conceptualising the measurement of health and disability. Its basic tenets have formed the rubric for PRO measures in a wide variety of health topics, including voice and voice disorders (Jacobson *et al.*, 1997; Hogikyan and Sethuraman, 1999). It is important to note that although it does provide a conceptual framework, it does not provide guidance on how to develop a PRO measure. Increased focus on patient-centred outcomes research has resulted in a proliferation of PRO measures with reportedly variable psychometric rigour (Johnston *et al.*, 2015).

Voice quality

Although the author is not in any way advocating that clinicians rely on value judgements without supporting acoustic data, for many experienced clinicians it is quite possible to make satisfactory judgements on vocal quality as a preliminary assessment measure. It is, however, worth noting that perceptual rating of voice quality is difficult and can be beset with difficulties not related to listener perception but to task design. Kreiman *et al.* (2007) explored when and why reliability is an issue of task design, not of listener unreliability, although it was noted that listeners achieved significantly better when assessing quality on a continuous versus a six-point scale. Kreiman and Gerratt (2011) continue to look at methods for reducing variability in voice quality measurements and conclude that aver-aging multiple ratings and standardising the mean are inadequate in addressing variations in voice quality perception.

Resonance

In assessing resonance the clinician is listening for an indication of faulty vocal resonance, principally the presence of hypernasality, hyponasality, cul-de-sac resonance or indeed a thin voice quality that lacks resonance. For this assessment the patient should be asked to read a standard passage, as already recommended for use in assessing habitual pitch, and the clinician should rate the severity of the hypernasality. It is important to assess the patient using connected speech as patients may not always demonstrate hypernasality on single words. It is also important to note any nasal escape of air. Reading a standard passage will also indicate the presence of hyponasality (where there is a lack of nasal res-onance when nasal consonants are phonated). It is also possible to ask the patient to hum and assess this. Most patients with hyponasality are unable to hum or at least unable to hum clearly. Cul-de-sac resonance is noted when the tongue is retracted and bunched in the oral cavity and appears to prevent a balance between oral and nasal resonance. A very thin vocal quality that is not related to a high pitch level is often related to an omission of oral resonance on vowel sounds, along with a high front of tongue position. This can be assessed by contrasting the vocal resonance achieved when producing velar consonants and back vowels to that of continuous speech. These, as with so many of the assessments already mentioned, are strongly dependent on the clinician's perceptual listener judgement. See GRBAS (Hirano, 1981) above. For that reason it is very important that clinicians, as noted in Chapter 4, periodically review their perceptual skills, perhaps with members of their clinical team or, if working on their own, with colleagues from other voice departments, in order to confirm that these skills remain well-honed and accurate. It is perhaps useful to echo the words of Kreiman *et al.* (1993) still relevant today:'In order for perceptual ratings to be useful, the listener or rater must use his/her set of internal references consistently'.

The assessment procedures outlined above, in addition to those details carefully amassed during the data gathering which built the patient profile, will give a useful overall subjective record of the patient's performance on certain tasks. It should be remembered that these tasks all offer perceptual information and by their very nature are not objective. This does not, however, reduce their assessment value and, in addition to results from instrumental evaluation of voice production through laryngeal endoscopic imaging, acoustic and aero-dynamic methods, are critical to management and treatment protocols.

Instrumentation

A multidimensional protocol was established by the European Laryngological Society (ELS) in order to reach better agreement and standardisation for functional assessment of patho-logic voices. The experiences of six European voice centres were analysed in a retrospective study in order to evaluate the validity, practicability and applicability of the protocol which comprised five dimensions: perceptual voice evaluation, videostroboscopy, acoustics, aero-dynamics and subjective rating by the patient (Dejonkere *et al.*, 2001). However, it proved difficult to ensure measurement consistency/repeatability and so individual countries and institutions appear to focus more on individual protocols, although all are agreed on the basic tenets of what needs to be assessed. In the USA, a recommended protocol for instru-mental assessment of vocal function was developed by an expert panel (Patel *et al.*, 2018) and it is to be recommended, as is the ASHA website offer (www.asha.org).

Essential measures required by the clinician for assessment purposes relate to acoustic, vibratory and aerodynamic features in addition to muscle action events. For the purposes of this chapter these assessment features will be looked at individually but with the recognition that a careful examination of all the information available leads to a differential diagnosis. Although objective assessment is part of the clinician's tool kit, the results obtained should be balanced by other factors, such as the information obtained from the case history and the perceptual assessment.

Commercially available equipment provides a number of different acoustic measurements. However, in this increasingly sophisticated market, instrumentation changes and develops not in a matter of years but rather months, so for that reason this section offers an overview of those vocal parameters that can be assessed, rather than attempting in any way to offer a list of equipment and equipment manufacturers. The choice of instrumentation will be dependent on budgetary and financial constraints, the expertise and experience of the clinical staff and the setting within which they are working; be that in, for example, a voice clinic or independently in a hospital setting with onward referrals from the ENT department.

Fundamental frequency

Fundamental frequency (of which the perceptual correlate is pitch) is an acoustic measurement recorded in hertz (Hz) that directly reflects the vibrating rate of the vocal folds. The assessment of fundamental frequency can be done in a variety of ways, the simplest being through sustained vowel phonation, where the patient is asked to sustain a vowel at a comfortable pitch and loudness level for a reasonable period of time. The disadvantage of this is that for many patients sustained phonation is difficult to achieve and so the use of a standard reading passage, as previously discussed, is a better solution.

Perturbation measures jitter and shimmer, and signal-to-noise ratios are frequently used to confirm perceptual judgements of quality deviation. Perturbation refers to the changes in the mass, tension and biomechanical characteristics of the vocal folds. Perturbation must be measured from sustained vowel production at a steady pitch level. Jitter, or short-term frequency variation, is obtained by measuring the period of each cycle of vibration, subtracting it from the previous or succeeding period, averaging the differences and dividing it by the average period. A common method of recording jitter is to establish a percentage figure of variation from cycle to cycle. For speakers with normal voices, jitter is expected to be below 1%, while in pathological voices and in some normal elderly voices, jitter ratio measurements are higher. Amplitude perturbation, or shimmer, refers to small cycle-to-cycle changes of the amplitude of the vocal fold signal, in other words short-term instability of the intensity of the vocal signal, and is measured in the same way as jitter, but usually reported in decibels (dB). Normative values for shimmer are usually in the range of 0.5–1.00 dB (Deem and Miller, 2000).

However, it is important to stress that it is difficult to be precise about norms for acoustic measures as there are many factors that mitigate all encompassing norms. These may relate to issues such as gender and age differences, cultural issues related to country norms and nationality and, most importantly, the testing environment to incorporate variation in the equipment and the use of different algorithms in the software used. Maryn *et al.* (2009), for example, compared jitter and shimmer measures using both the Multi-Dimensional Voice Program with Praat programs and concluded that 'one can hardly compare frequency perturbation across systems and programs and amplitude perturbation outcomes across systems'.

Moreover, it should be noted that amplitude and pitch perturbations must be combined with other voice parameters for assessment and it would be unwise to rely on one or two measures alone, although in terms of measuring and monitoring change or improvement they are useful markers. As with any outcome measures, true validation of change comes from using before and after case study design with the same equipment, so mitigating uncertainty.

Frequency range measurement (the range of frequencies from highest to lowest that the patient can produce) reflects the physiological limits of the patient's voice and can be measured in hertz or semi-tones by any of the equipment previously mentioned or by the phonetogram. The phonetogram is increasingly considered to be part of the standardised test battery in Europe, providing measures of sound intensity and frequency. Sound spectrograms reflect the vibratory characteristics of the vocal folds and the vocal tract, and are useful not only for analysing but also for showing change in the spectral characteristics of the sound at the level of the vocal folds. Spectrograms provide harmonics-to-noise ratio or signal-to-noise ratio measures. This provides a measure of the frequencies produced by the vibrating vocal folds or the energy in the harmonics of the voice signal and the noise energy in the signal.

With voice disorders there is commonly greater noise and less energy in the harmonics of the sound, hence the term 'harmonics-to-noise ratio'. Distortion and variation in harmonics give clues to the degree of distortion occurring to vocal-fold vibration. Sophisticated computerised speech laboratories are available which can offer a number of options.

These must be considered within the resources available and the needs of the department. Some computer programs such as Praat (Boersma, 2001) mentioned above are available for analysing, synthesising and manipulating speech and other sounds, and for creating publication-quality graphics. It is open source and available free of charge for all major computer platforms. It can be downloaded from www.praat.org.

Vibratory features

Laryngographic measurement of the vocal folds offers qualitative and quantitative information on the entire phase of the vocal fold vibratory cycle. The Lx waveform produced may be displayed on an oscilloscope or visual display unit providing instantaneous feedback for the clinician and the patient. As a therapeutic tool it is very helpful to see both the shape of the waveform and how it changes pre- and post-therapy. Electroglottography (EGG) is a non-invasive technique for recording the time cycle of glottal opening and closing movements of the vocal folds during phonation. Boehme and Gross (2005) suggest that the EGG can be used to determine fundamental frequency, recognise periodicity, assess voice register, determine the speed of vocal-fold closure, assess voice onset and build-up, assess hyperfunction and hypofunction and as a biofeedback method. Operating on the basis of a constant voltage monitoring of translaryngeal electrical conductance, monitoring is by means of guard ring electrodes applied to the skin superficial to each wing of the thyroid cartilage. When the soft tissue area of the vocal folds is in full contact, maximum conductance is recorded – shown on the screen as the peak of the waveform. When no contact is made, minimum conductance is recorded – the trough of the waveform. The leading edge of the waveform gives a precise indication of the beginning of the closure phase. With a portable laryngograph the Lx waveform can be recorded with speech on one channel and Lx on the other, then viewed on the oscilloscope or programmed into a computer for display or printout, giving acoustic and vibratory features at the same time.

Stroboscopy

Stroboscopic examination provides precise information on the vocal folds at different phases in their vibratory cycle. The shape and condition of the free edges, the shape of the glottis and supraglottis, and, particularly useful, the vibration of the vocal folds in slow motion can be monitored. The stroboscope is in effect an electronic light source which can be synchronised with that of a vibrating or rotating object. Detailed examination under continuous lighting is impossible by the naked eye due to the speed of the movement. Because the intermittent light occurs at a frequency just slightly less than the rate of actual fold vibration at any given time, the eye perceives a slow-motion movement. It is also possible to see the vibration pattern of the vocal folds plus the mucosal wave and to determine if this is symmetrical. If the frequency of the intermittent light flash is synchronised with the frequency of vocal-fold movement then it will always be illuminated in the same phase of its cycle, appearing to be motionless. Videostroboscopy allows the clinician to make a permanent record of the vocal-fold vibratory patterns which may be used to monitor progress and treatment outcome measures. It also allows the clinician to capture data which can be sent to the patient's GP. Videostroboscopy training is available to clinicians as many clinicians with a voice specialism now routinely examine their own patients as part of their intervention. Procedures differ in different settings, but it is usual for clinicians to have the option to discuss findings with ENT colleagues, although this is not always the case. It should be noted that although stroboscopy offers a factual record, interpretation is subjective, so clinicians may interpret the same information differently. It should be remembered that any assessment, irrespective of how sophisticated, is a measure of a moment in time.

Summary

The multi-faceted approach to voice assessment examined in this and the preceding chapter has looked at the nature of information gathering for the diagnosis and differential diagnosis of voice disorders. Information is drawn from the patient's case history, which explored through self-reporting the patient's medical history, the nature of the change in the sound of the voice, the pitch, extent and volume of the voice, voice quality change and its severity and episodes of voice loss. Pitch range, onset of the note, volume, respiratory control, nasality and stability is provided through auditory perceptual evaluation. Data providing objective measures are gained from acoustic analyses, aerodynamic and vibratory measures in addition to the classic assessment of the laryngeal structures and visualisation of vocal-fold vibration by means of instrumentation. Undoubtedly, the exponential increase in technology will allow for increasing sophistication in the availability and use of new instrumentation by clinicians in the coming years (Francis *et al.*, 2017). Notwithstanding an increasing battery of assessment tools, the skills of the clinician will still be paramount in the perceptual assessment and treatment of the voice patient.

TREATMENT AND MANAGEMENT STRATEGIES

Introduction

Having completed the patient profile and fulfilled all the necessary assessment procedures, the clinician should have a clear view of the patient's current vocal status and in consultation with the patient agreed a plan for the future. For that reason the use of SOAP notes to confirm that nothing germane to a successful clinical outcome has been omitted or overlooked is recommended. The patient's file should contain the following information:

> *S*ubjective results – gained from information such as historical data, patient symptoms, the patient's perceptions and reports of events.
> *O*bjective results – gained from measurable, quantifiable and observable information.
> *A*ssessment results – gained from interpretation of these subjective and objective data.
> *P*lan – based upon the continuing assessment of new data and of the intervention in general; plans for intervention may be changed or modified.

Well-written SOAP notes convey the actions of the clinician and the response of the patient. In essence, SOAP notes provide an answer to the question 'What did the clinician do and how did the patient respond?' Using SOAP notes is a useful and pragmatic way to ensure that treatment strategies are well-considered and well thought through. It allows the clinician to confirm, for example, that the need for further diagnostic work or new therapeutic plans has been considered and provides proof that an activity was completed in the case of future audit, conflict or litigation. The adage 'if it wasn't documented, it wasn't done' is very relevant in the case of SOAP notes. In addition, depending on each individual situation, the clinician can confirm that the patient's family and, in some cases, work colleagues are fully 'on-board' in terms of intervention and if not, what, if any, additional support needs to be put in place. SOAP notes may also be used along with various outcome measures which will be discussed later in the chapter. It is, however, possible to keep to concise note-taking while fulfilling the requirements of outcome measures and SOAP notes, without extensive paperwork. The acronym ACUTE, standing for Accurate, Codeable, Understandable, Timely and Error-free is a useful way to check SOAP notes, in fact a useful acronym for any record taking. Multiple systems exist to handle SOAP notes and there is therapy documentation software available to keep track of SOAP notes, but these provisions will obviously be dependent on what is available within individual workplaces. It is helpful to remember that SOAP notes are designed to assist rather than overwhelm the intervention process.

While this approach is clinically robust it is important to remember that in certain instances the ideal is not always easily achieved. For example, funding restrictions may prevent access to objective assessment resources or to further phonosurgery or psychological services, or indeed the patient may present with a complex disorder that requires a number of interventions. Despite this, however, the clinician can be encouraged by the fact that voice therapy has been shown to be effective with a number of different voice disorders (Dejardins *et al.*, 2016; Carding *et al.*, 2017) and clinicians do have access to many different treatment strategies which can effect change in voice disorders.

This chapter will look at aspects of intervention which should be considered alongside strategic management choices. In the author's view, treatment and management strategies should be thought of as a continuum and, as was described above, SOAP notes allow for modification of both treatment and strategic plans. Practical voice exercises, which it is hoped clinicians will find useful, and other treatment programmes and approaches are provided in Chapter 7.

Intervention: interdependence of a number of factors

An important consideration for the clinician in treatment planning must be how to evaluate, predict, monitor and measure outcomes in an episode of care. Treatment efficacy and effectiveness is increasingly important in terms of therapy outcomes, but so too is the need to make sure that the proposed intervention will best fit the patient. Consideration of a care pathway should, as has already been discussed, always incorporate those aspects of the WHO's International Classification of Functioning, Disability and Health (ICF; WHO, 2001), which provides a model of human functioning and disability, as well as a classification system that allows for all dimensions of disability to be highlighted and measured, including voice disorders. ICF describes how people live with their health condition. Because an individual's functioning and disability occurs in a context, ICF also includes a list of environmental factors. ICF provides a useful biopsychosocial framework to understand and measure health outcomes and can be used in clinical settings, health services or surveys at the individual or population level. Thus, ICF complements ICD-10, the International Statistical Classification of Diseases and Related Health Problems (WHO, 2008), and looks beyond mortality and disease. In this way it allows comparability with other health conditions as well as evaluation of the role of the environment as a cause of disability among people with voice disorders. It is recognised that our knowledge of voice disorder-related burden is incomplete and it is certainly important to add to it through epidemiological studies. Even if this approach is not used in full, it is important for the clinician to consider how a patient with a voice disorder may have difficulty functioning within a particular environment and how disabling this is. It is also important to consider the patient's well-being in terms of the amount of distress, anxiety, passivity or positive adjustment a patient expresses regarding their vocal diagnosis. This may range from anxiety and stress about maintaining current employment to appearing inadequate and being embarrassed by vocal inconsistency. It could also be a response to the reactions of others and the degree of perceived support and encouragement which the patient experiences. Well-being and distress are dependent on such variable factors and can differ greatly from one person to another. A similar disorder in two patients may lead to a minimal loss of well-being in one but severe emotional disturbance in another. Similarly, what may appear to be a minimal disturbance in voice quality may be of little significance to one patient but a major problem to an occupational voice user in the elite performer category. The necessity to evaluate patients holistically and to plan treatment and management strategies accordingly, acknowledging the interdependence of many different factors, is of paramount importance and is the author's preferred approach. For example, when patients are distressed, it is likely that posture and movement may be affected. Similarly, patients who have attended for daily radiotherapy may feel unwell, exhausted and have continuing anxiety regarding their current or future health status, which may result in muscle tension dysphonia and inhibition of maximal improvement.

Starting all treatment planning with a whole-person, goal-orientated, 'Person-centred care' approach means that patients' values and preferences are sought and, once expressed, guide all aspects of their health care, supporting their realistic health and life goals. The American Geriatrics Society expert panel on person-centred care suggests that 'Person-centred care is achieved through a dynamic relationship among individuals, others who are important to them, and all relevant providers. This collaboration informs decision-making to the extent that the individual desires' (2015). Thus, all aspects of treatment goals and their application can be examined and assessed so that intervention is then based not only on the known and specific relationship of treatment approaches to aspects of voice physiology, but also targeted to the specific presenting disorder of the patient in partnership with the clinician and the patient's family if appropriate.

Person-centred functional goals maximise outcomes that are important to the individual, and to this end the author's approach is to build voice work on a strong foundation. This foundation comprises 'building blocks' of posture, alignment, release of tension/relaxation and breathing, with voice, pitch and muscular flexibility providing a second tier, followed by the final tier of resonance. This, however, is a personal choice and it is for that reason that the exercises in the next chapter follow that prescription in terms of their ordering. It is readily acknowledged that an experienced clinician can identify where a patient has a particular problem and voice work can be targeted specifically. This targeted approach is, however, not always helpful for the inexperienced clinician, who may not have had sufficient clinical practice to recognise the absence of such critical building blocks and so fail to direct the patient to invest in the required preparatory stages.

Achieving lasting change

Voice therapy should, if possible, be seen by patients as a process of effecting permanent vocal change, rather than as a way of achieving vocal change through a series of exercises which they 'do' or 'do not do'. Patients need to recognise that voice therapy is not analogous to some forms of medication – 'Take three times a day and expect improvement' – but to see it rather as a process which takes considerable effort of, by, for and with both clinician and patient, in addition to constant monitoring to achieve results. In effecting change it is, in the author's view, important that recognition is given to aspects that underpin the relationship between both patient and clinician and which may affect intervention and treatment outcomes, for example, individual learning styles, clinical skills, compliance, tacit knowledge, reflection and learning modalities. Theories of learning styles abound, suggesting that individuals learn best if the information given is targeted to the learning style/ability of the individual. That said, some results challenge the hypothesis that individuals learn best with material presented in a particular sensory modality (Krätzig and Arbuthnott, 2006). Willingham *et al.* (2015) suggest that individuals can have a preference for processing certain types of information or for processing information in certain types of ways. By understanding that individual patients can have quite different learning preferences the clinician can adopt effective communication strategies such as privileging a visual over an auditory approach when delivering information; it is certainly worth being open to the idea of learning preferences.

Clinical skills

Development of clinical skills is enhanced by opportunities for clinicians to observe different clinical settings. Funding and training opportunities may well restrict interested clinicians from following up on those opportunities for continuing professional development. However, for newly qualified and less-experienced clinicians it is important for learning to have an explicit framework which spotlights the decisions that experienced and effective clinicians make instinctively and implicitly. In framing future intervention decisions, questions which require a clinically reasoned response are very useful. The following are included with permission of the then Professional Studies Team, at City, University of London (2010):

1   Is there a need for SLT involvement?
2   What is the nature of the SLT difficulty?
3   Does it warrant SLT involvement?
4   When would SLT services no longer be warranted?
5   What is the ultimate goal of therapy?
6   What service delivery would be most effective in achieving this goal?
7   What is the episode of care goal?
8   How can this goal be achieved outside the clinical context?
9   How is change going to be measured?
10   What is the sequence of session goals that lead to the attainment of the episode of care goal?
11   How are the session goals going to be implemented?
12   How does outcome affect future management of the patient?

The therapeutic relationship

No matter how expert a clinician may be, the therapeutic process will not advance if the patient does not engage in it. Here the issues of compliance, adherence, concordance, tacit knowledge and reflection need to be examined. Usually seen within a medicinal pre-scribing regime, the author proposes that the concept of patient engagement should be widened into investigating how intervention may be affected by the patient's belief in the clinician's recommended treatment plan and how the patient can 'buy' into it for long-term success. Compliance is defined as the extent to which the patient's behaviour matches the prescriber's recommendations. This is not, however, a particularly useful term, as it implies a lack of patient involvement in the decision-making process. Adherence is defined as the extent to which the patient's behaviour matches agreed recommendations from the prescriber. This is a term adopted by many as an alternative to compliance in an attempt to emphasise that the patient is free to decide whether to adhere to the doctor's recommendations and that failure to do so should not be a reason to blame the patient. Concordance is a relatively recent term predominately used in the United Kingdom and its definition is that of a concept which stretches from prescribing communication to patient support in medicine taking.

For the clinician working with a voice patient it is important to recognise that progress will succeed long-term only if there is concordance between clinician and patient as intervention is no longer paternalistic but is more person-centred, whole-person 'option'-driven. Clearly the process towards achieving lasting vocal change involves a multiplicity of factors and requires a raft of clinical skills, many of which develop over time and with experience. In light of these many and varied approaches, perhaps it is helpful to mention that individual preferences in therapy techniques are not only acceptable but inevitable. Some styles of therapy will suit some clinicians and be quite appropriate to their natural therapy style. In the author's opinion two significant, widely used and successful approaches applied to voice disorders are cognitive-behavioural therapy (CBT; Butcher *et al.*, 2007) and solution-focused brief therapy (SFBT; Burns, 2016; Burns and Northcott, 2021). Training in both these approaches is essential before they become part of the clinician's toolkit, but they are worth exploring further and very much allow clinicians to meet the philosophy of providing patient-centred care.

In terms of voice disorders with a psychological bias (as discussed in Chapter 2), Butcher *et al.* suggest that CBT has relevance because it is a model that can be used to teach ways of managing anxiety and lowered mood, to train patients in communication and social interaction skills and in life management skills. The central principle of CBT is that the ways in which an individual behaves are determined by the individual's interpretations of himself and the situations he encounters. Therefore, CBT takes account of how emotional, psychosocial and biophysical processes shape behaviour. The individual is helped to make sense of experiences as well as how cognitions (thoughts and images) affect both emotions and behaviour. Through increased self-knowledge the individual learns he has the potential for personal change and development.

Solution-focused brief therapy is a type of talking therapy that is based upon social constructionist philosophy. It focuses on what patients want to achieve through therapy, rather than on the problem(s) that made them seek help. The approach focuses on past successes as well as future descriptions of the client's desired outcome. The therapist uses respectful curiosity to invite the patient to envisage their preferred future and then the clinician and patient start attending to any moves towards it, whether these are small, incremental or large changes. To support this, questions are asked about the patient's story, strengths and resources, and about exceptions to the problem.

Solution-focused therapists believe that change is constant. By helping people identify the things that they wish to change in their life and those things that they wish to continue to happen, SFBT therapists help their patients to construct a concrete vision of a preferred future for themselves. The SFBT clinician then helps the patient to identify times in their current life that are closer to this future and examines what is different on these occasions. By bringing these small successes to their awareness and helping them repeat the successful things they do when the problem is not there or is less severe, the clinician helps the patient move towards the preferred future they have identified.

Tacit knowledge is a construct conceived by Polanyi (1967), who wrote that we should start from the fact that 'we can know more than we can tell', terming this pre-logical phase of knowing as 'tacit knowledge'. Tacit knowledge comprises a range of conceptual and sensory information and images that can be brought to bear in an attempt to make sense of something. Translating this into clinical practice, Polanyi's concept of a tacit dimension allows clinicians to value intuition and hunches, and come to a better understanding of what is going on in certain situations. This may well encourage clinicians to feel confident that their tacit knowledge is of value in the face of a concern over reasoned and critical interrogation. It may also allow clinicians to better understand that a patient's resistance to a particular intervention, despite evidence to the contrary, may be due to their pre-existing tacit knowledge.

Schon (1983) was a pioneer in bringing reflection into the centre of professional practice and the notion of reflection in action and on action is an important aspect of intervention, allowing the clinician to think on their feet but at the same time look at a situation about which some uncertainty exists, and connect it to their previous experience. This online thinking is important and may not relate to textbook examples. Reflecting on action happens after the event or the encounter, when the clinician examines why they acted as they did and what happened as a result of their actions. In this way a clinician can build up a portfolio of images, ideas, examples and actions that they can draw upon. For the inexperienced clinician these portfolios are embryonic and not always adequate in terms of dealing with patients. Without the security of reflection both in- and on-action it may be difficult to find evidence to present to a patient in terms of how to deal with a particular impasse. Reflective practice is key to the development of professional practice, but it is important to also consider that in fulfilling the demands of evidence-based clinical practice and therapy outcome measures, there could be an inherent danger in that it may limit the influence and reduce the value of the highly important role of experiential knowledge in clinical work (Butler, 2019). It could also reduce the focus and influence of qualitative research within voice therapy, which would, in the author's opinion, be most unfortunate as the role of the clinician when working with voice patients is similar to that of the researcher who works within the qualitative paradigm. An underlying assumption of the qualitative paradigm involves the relationships of the researcher and the researched. Because researchers are part of the reality they study, their neutrality is impossible and their goal is to be aware and conscious of their biases and prejudices and to monitor them through the processes of data collection and analysis. This is a process which, in the author's opinion, is very similar to the way in which the clinician engages with the voice patient, establishing the facts through ethnographic and phenomenological interviewing, examining personal prejudices and biases and monitoring them through case history and assessment data to arrive at shaping influences and value patterns in the therapeutic process, leading to a successful outcome. This is why it is so important to have opportunities for reflection, supervision and opportunities for continuing professional development at every stage in a career.

In considering the roles and responsibilities of clinician and patient in terms of intervention and management, it is important to look at the critical issue of patient responsibility. Much of the patient's voice use will be outside the clinic and for that reason time spent on managing this aspect is very important. However, the clinician also has a responsibility to ensure that the voice work that has been done in clinic is sufficiently robust to underpin and support the voice in the variety of speaking environments in which patients are placed and in which they try to function. Vocal competence within the clinical setting is rarely fully tested. The nature of voice therapy is that the clinician's aim is to offer a safe vocal environment which allows patients to explore their vocal boundaries and try to achieve change. This safe environment, while clinically desirable, does have the more negative effect of never really replicating the vocally challenging situations which have often contributed to the voice disorder in the first place. Is it necessary to replicate these challenging situations? Is it not sufficient to simply achieve consistent vocal change within the clinic and assume that this will allow the patient to 'cope' with the challenges of voice use outside this rather protected environment? As noted earlier, studies have proved that voice therapy is effective but it is, in the author's opinion, also necessary to test this effectiveness by 'challenging' the voice. Then the clinician is, in fact, fully meeting the requirements of successful voice therapy outcome measures. It could also be said that it is of inestimable value for patients to have the opportunity to explore how their voice functions when challenged. In addition, it ensures that patients do not feel vulnerable when faced with a similar experience once therapy has been completed. Faced with the exigencies of the National Health Service in the United Kingdom, clinicians may feel that the time and resources needed to oversee this approach make it unrealistic. Indeed, health insurance provision in other countries is also increasingly restrictive, but the author would argue that this approach does in fact reduce the likelihood of the patient returning subsequently for further therapy. So how does one ensure that patients are well prepared for all potential speaking situations outside the clinic? What are the clinical considerations? Are there certain checks and balances that the clinician can undertake to ensure that the patient is prepared for the unexpected, before treatment is completed?

The following issues are presented for consideration.

Competence in the clinic

Competence in the clinic is not always a guarantee of success. Readers will have experience of patients who have appeared to achieve excellent voice use in the clinical setting but who are unable to achieve the same level of competence away from this safe environment or, indeed, away from the clinician. While it may be flattering to feel that it is 'our' influence which allows a patient to succeed, treatment which promotes too much reliance by the patient on the individual clinician cannot be deemed a success.

Monitor patients in their work and social environment

The clinician needs to ensure that clinical competence is achieved by the patient away from the safety of the clinical environment. The increasing sophistication of mobile technology will allow the clinician a 'virtual' view of a patient in their place of work or home environment, in order to assess and monitor their physical environment and voice use. This would obviously be subject to proper rigour in terms of data protection issues, but it is worth a discussion with the patient. This 'virtual tour' could then prompt a discussion regarding changes that could be introduced in an effort, for example, to promote better posture or arrange their work station more ergonomically, if appropriate. Similarly performers can either record themselves or ask someone to record their own performances in order to allow the clinician to assess volume and projection and get a much more accurate representation of the vocal demands that the patient experiences and to note much more clearly any episodes of vocal misuse.

Speaking under stress

Patients often report that the greatest challenge to their voice is when speaking under stress. If the patient is able to predict these episodes then treatment strategies can be successful. For example, with difficult work-related issues patients may be able to prepare vocally for these encounters. Close relationship difficulties relating to domestic and highly emotional situations are the most difficult to anticipate, and indeed it is the physiological response to the emotion of the situation which jeopardises the best vocal preparation, for example, increased heart rate, shallow breathing or pharyngeal constriction. It is, however, possible to offer patients strategies for dealing with them by, for example, reducing sentence length, limiting pharyngeal constriction and minimising hard attack. (Exercises for these are to be found in Chapter 7.)

Meeting the vocal challenge

Presenting patients with these challenges while still in therapy allows them time to explore ways of dealing with them effectively. While therapy must at all times promote self-awareness and self-monitoring, it must also present the patient with challenges. In meeting these challenges, patients can overcome any residual fear that, once away from the safety of the clinic, vocal dangers are ready to deracinate all achievement to date. Patients can then confidently accept responsibility for self-management, the ultimate aim of any inter-vention. The acid test of the success of any clinical intervention must be whether the indi-vidual acquires the ability to monitor their voice on an ongoing basis, learning to recognise and accurately predict situations that are potentially vocally abusive. The clinician must encourage this skill and also ensure that patients are fully aware of the various factors that influence vocal performance.

The occupational voice user

It is imperative that intervention offers occupational voice users skills to maintain voice even when severely vocally challenged, providing them with strategies to monitor their own voice and recognise factors that may precipitate vocal misuse. This approach may be pre-referral or preventative in nature; for example, clinicians may offer probationer teacher workshops in conjunction with education departments or as part of Initial Teacher Training. (A sample programme is offered at the end of Chapter 7.) Voice boot camps (Patel *et al.*, 2011), where treatment is highly concentrated for short periods, lasting up to a week, are now considered highly efficacious, but clearly this option is subject to a number of issues defined by the organisation within which a clinician is working. The success of any pro-gramme of intervention depends on the individual's ability to generalise techniques into their working environment. It is also imperative to build on what has been learned within the supportive clinical environment to achieve effective voice use at all times that will allow the occupational voice user to return to, and retain, their professional role at all times.

The voice review checklist

As noted above, patients spend the majority of their time away from clinical supervision. It is therefore very important to try to encourage patients to systematically and objectively examine how they use their voice and to monitor their vocal quality during that time, thus engendering a shared sense of responsibility in effecting change. In order to do this consist-ently, the author recommends the use of the Voice Review Checklist. Appendix III provides a hard copy which may be photocopied. It may be used during therapy so that patients can use the information to review how they have been feeling and what, if any, changes they note that affect their voice during a specific time period. This information may then be shared with the clinician on subsequent appointments. Post-intervention, patients may continue to use the Voice Review Checklist to ensure that they remain focused and aware of any change in vocal quality. A simple tick list response is all that is required, but it does offer an 'at-a-glance' check as to changes in vocal quality, evidence of symptoms such as tiredness, stress and illness and elements in their working environment that are giving cause for concern: for example, they may report that their working environment is very poorly ventilated, or that it is very dry and hot with poor acoustics. One section allows the patient to indicate strategies they have used to maintain their voice, such as vocal rest, steaming or limiting their time in noisy environments. Work is ongoing on a Voice Review Checklist App which should further streamline the process.

Another useful resource is the *Voice Diary* which is reproduced in Appendix IV. This allows identification of the periods of most vocal loading during the week and will highlight those periods during which vocal recovery could take place. As well as examining this aspect of voice use it is also possible to encourage patients to try to pre-empt periods of potential vocal danger, so increasing their own self-awareness. One of the most effective ways in which this may be done is to divide the week into units of time (morning, afternoon and evening are suggested) and to use the following headings: voice rest, easy voicing, vocal stress, vocal loading. It may seem rather prescriptive to suggest that a chart is completed, but the visual representation does, in fact, provide much more focus for the patient. A visual representation of the week showing periods of high voice use juxtaposed, it is hoped, with periods of voice rest or easy voicing is very illuminating for the patient. Despite ensuring that opportunities for questions and discussion of any issues of concern are built into appointment sessions, clinicians are always aware of the need to seek confirmation that the information given has been clearly understood and assimilated. This can offer useful insight into the patient's real understanding of specific contributory factors and allow the clinician to clarify any misunderstanding and reinforce advice. For example, when looking at the week ahead, a patient may correctly identify a high level of vocal stress related to, for example, attendance at a family party. There may not be the same recognition that taking children to the swimming baths can be just as vocally stressful, due to the acoustics of the swimming baths, which can often affect the patient's auditory perceptual ability and so encourage overly forced voicing. Although it is not always possible to accurately predict events for a week ahead, most individuals will have some knowledge of their likely activities. Once some pattern emerges, then it is possible to help the patient to 'manage' periods of vocal stress. If it is not possible to alter or adjust weekly activities, then at least the clinician should try to encourage periods of vocal recovery after heavy voice use. While a patient's vocal stress may be identified, as illustrated above, it is important for the clinician to be aware of the link between voice and stress and to remember that stress and issues of stress increasingly feature in many patients' lives.

Stress

In any discussion of stress it is important to try to define what is understood by the term 'stress' and that in itself can be a problem, as tension, strain and pressure are words that can be used synonymously with 'stress'. Stress can be seen paradoxically as both negative and positive. It affects everyone, but not to the same extent. Recent research shows that work-related stress can affect anyone at any level, it is not confined to those with, for example, heavy occupational responsibilities. Stress is not an illness – it is a state. There is a difference between pressure and stress. Pressure can be positive and a motivating factor that is often essential in a job as it helps individuals to achieve their goals and perform better, but when the demands of the work are perceived by an individual as greater than their ability to cope, stress is experienced. Stress occurs as a natural reaction to too much pressure, but it also provides a necessary and essential warning sign of impending danger or that something is wrong.

In the UK a government agency, the Health and Safety Executive (HSE), recorded figures for 2018/19 of 602,000 people who were off work suffering from stress, depression or anxiety and 12.8 million working days were lost due to work-related stress, depression and anxiety. Similar figures can be found globally. The European Agency for Safety and Health at Work noted that in 34 countries, the education and health sectors were one of the most affected sectors. So when working with Occupational Voice Users, the majority of whom, historically, will be teachers and lecturers, it is important to recognise that stress is a considerable element in their work. It should also be noted that it is not only patients but clinicians that are also affected by stress. The number of prescriptions for antidepressants in England almost doubled in the decade from 2008 to 2018. Data from NHS Digital show that 70.9 million prescriptions for antidepressants were given out in 2018, compared with 36 million in 2008. The number has been steadily increasing year-on-year (*British Medical Journal*, 2019).

Shown below are some of the physiological changes that occur as the body, responding to the threat of stress, prepares for action by exciting the 'fight or flight' response and releasing cortisol, adrenaline and noradrenaline.

* difficulty in swallowing,
* aching neck,
* backache,

- muscle tension,
- muscle pain,
- fatigue,
- frequent urination and diarrhoea,
- less-efficient immune system,
- overbreathing,
- indigestion.

If these physical changes, which occur as a result of stress, are examined in the light of the processes that affect voice, then the link between voice and stress may be seen more clearly.

The following is offered as a brief résumé to better highlight the link for patients:

- difficulty in swallowing, from a dry mouth, may be associated with a fixed laryngeal position;
- an aching neck, from muscle tension, may lead to tension in the internal and external muscles of the larynx;
- backache, from the contraction of large skeletal muscles, affects the easy movement of the ribs resulting in a reduction in lung volume and breath support for the voice;
- muscle tension, similarly, reduces the flexibility and muscularity of the respiratory process;
- muscle pain leads to reduced volitional movement, leading to stiffness and loss of flexibility both of the ribs and the vocal folds;
- fatigue leads to loss of effective muscle function and a consequent reduction in the flexibility and easy movement of the vocal folds;
- frequent urination and diarrhoea lead to dehydration and a consequent effect on vocal quality;
- a compromised immune system leads to lowered resistance to upper respiratory tract infections and the potential for infection within the larynx, leading to changes in the mass of the vocal folds which in turn affects pitch and range;
- overly rapid breathing leads to a reduction in both breath support and phonation time. It may also cause hyperventilation, dizziness and light-headedness;
- indigestion may lead to gastro-oesophageal reflux, which will directly affect the vocal folds, causing inflammation and irritation and a change in the quality of the sound.

This very brief outline of the physiological changes demonstrates the far-reaching effects of stress on the voice. It can be seen to affect every aspect of phonation, from breath capacity to muscle function, reduced lubrication of the vocal folds to changes within the lining of the vocal tract and the tissue integrity of the vocal folds. Many patients find this information illuminating, as the link between stress and voice may not previously have been well signalled. While it is, of course, useful for the patient to make this link, there must also be recognition of the need to deal with whatever issues are giving rise to stress. Not to deal with stress may well militate against long-term therapeutic gain and it may be that the clinician is in a position to encourage change.

It is at all times important to remember that the perception of stress varies from individual to individual. For some, stress is a stimulating and exciting experience:they see the demands they face as challenging and feel in charge, so the consequent stress is good stress. Faced with the same situation, another individual will find the situation insupportable. Stress is a result of the individual's interpretation of the demands and their capabilities to cope, not the demands and capabilities themselves. Clinicians will also react individually to a patient's stress, so it is important not to offer specific advice but rather to offer strategies for achieving change.

The role of the clinician

Developing the range of skills and knowledge and/or experience of various interventions can prove daunting to an inexperienced clinician; indeed, the debate of who should treat the voice-disordered patient is a complex one which requires careful consideration. In reaching this decision, a variety of factors must be decided, including the available staffing resources, as well as providing a service for each patient which is equitable, based on best practice and/or evidence-based practice, and is of the highest quality available. In the UK, the Royal College of Speech and Language Therapists (RCSLT) provides considerable guidance for those in the UK and similarly, professional organisations in other countries will do the same, outlining a service model which should provide an equitable approach to all patients.

Staffing provision and distribution is determined by a number of factors, including financial resources, demand and the number of available staff at any given time. Malcomess (2005), in the *Core Care Aims Model* training programme, recommends that the most senior and specialised staff members, who have greatest experience and expertise, should be those spending most time on targeted services as this is most effective in prevention. It is to be hoped that where specialist clinicians are available, their remit must include training, encouraging and equipping the next generation of specialist therapists, some of this being accomplished by observation, shadowing, training and mentoring. In a fairly small specialty such as voice disorders, sharing of knowledge and expertise is paramount for the development and continuation of best practice and delivery of patient care.

Membership of Clinical Excellence Networks (CENs) where Speech and Language Therapists local to a region share the same area of interest and expertise is prominent in the UK. Clinicians usually meet several times during the year to share knowledge and develop their skills through study days. In the UK, the British Voice Association (BVA) has a reciprocal agreement with Voice CENs who circulate their members with information about BVA events and provide information about their study days. Similar networking and special interest group opportunities flourish in different countries.

The patient's perception and partnership

As we accept that clinicians will have differing approaches to intervention, so we must consider the patient's preferences and their perception of the whole intervention episode, their partnership role in the therapeutic intervention and their motivation to change. It was mentioned in an earlier chapter that it is not unusual for patients to express their confusion at referral to a voice clinic, and that this may also involve misunderstanding and a negative response. In addition, it must be acknowledged that cultural differences may lead patients to be concerned regarding discussion of personal matters, being observed or touched during therapy. It is important that the clinician attend an awareness session or study day on the importance of equality and diversity. Indeed, in many authorities this training is mandatory.

With this knowledge, the clinician should explain at all times the need for detailed personal information and the benefit or necessity of any physical contact, ensuring understanding and compliance by the patient. Similarly, the clinician should be extremely sensitive at all times to any possible misunderstanding, whether this arises from cultural, religious, ethnic or gender boundaries. On occasions, transfer to a clinician of a different culture, religion, ethnicity or gender may be preferred and should not be considered an admission of inadequacy or failure.

It is also necessary at the beginning of the care episode that patients are completely aware of the expectations of their role and participation in the therapy process. Some services provide a leaflet outlining the attendance and failure to attend policy, so that the patient is aware of the commitment required to undertake a course of voice therapy and the likely outcome of failing to attend. With an understanding of participation and partnership, goals can be established for the care episode with clarity of purpose for all parties.

Clinical effectiveness/clinical efficiencies

Clinical effectiveness, efficacy and efficiency have been at the forefront of clinicians' minds for many years with innumerable research and audit projects to evaluate various interventions, service delivery, quality and financial efficiency. This has become not only a feature of the voice clinician's awareness but impacts clinicians of all grades as well as their managers. Indeed, it is now necessary that all services have a specific means of monitoring and evaluating their service to provide regular reports on quality, clinical outcomes and efficiency so that equity of access, clinical effectiveness and financial efficiency can be demonstrated throughout the service. It is therefore necessary for services to select which-ever process suits best to address clinical judgement and reasoning, decision making and goal setting, while providing a workable means of monitoring on a daily basis. Three fre-quently used processes are the Care Aims Framework (Malcomess, 2005, 2015), Therapy Outcome Measures (TOMs; Enderby and John, 2015, 2019) and SMART goals, although there are many others. The three outlined below have different philosophies, cultures and uses within a clinical setting but fulfil synergistic roles.

The Care Aims philosophy is not a model of practice but is instead an overarching reasoning and decision-making framework. It is not used to describe inputs and outputs but rather reasoned predicted outcomes. Malcomess describes it as based on the assumption that 'as public services we have a fundamental duty to do the most good and the least harm for the most number of people within the resources available. The only equitable way of doing this is by working out who is most at risk in our population and which of those people we can help most' (Malcomess, 2005). Helping the population manage its own risk is at the heart of the approach, as is sound clinical judgement, reasoning and clinical decision making. It is impact-based, following the decision-making loop of identifying the impact or future impact of the problem, disorder or situation and the ability of the clinician to address this. Goals are set for intervention based on the impact and clinical effectiveness measured by reviewing the impact. The level of need is assessed, using the same clinical skills, and a decision reached on the level of input which is necessary for the patient. Any clinicians using this approach must attend the requisite training in Care Aims.

Therapy Outcome Measures (TOMs) measure four dimensions on a rating scale according to the clinician's clinical judgement. The four dimensions originate in the International Classification of Functioning, Disability and Health (ICF; WHO, 2001), mentioned earlier in this chapter and which is the framework for measuring health and disability advocated by the World Health Organization. 'By shifting the focus from cause to impact it places all health conditions on an equal footing allowing them to be compared using a common metric – the ruler of health and disability. Furthermore ICF takes into account the social aspects of disability and does not see disability only as a "medical" or "biological" dysfunction' (WHO, 2008). The dimensions listed below with voice examples are from a benchmarking study to compare outcomes of voice services specifically in the United Kingdom (John *et al.*, 2005). They are:

- Impairment (the degree of severity of the voice disorder).
- Disability/activity (the degree of limitation in use of voice).
- Handicap/participation (amount of disadvantage to social participation).
- Well-being of the patient (effect on emotion/level of distress).

TOMs are widely used in many disorders by many health professionals. As with Care Aims, it is recommended that staff receive training in this approach before using the outcome measures. The measurement of the outcomes associated with speech and language therapy is an essential component of delivering effective and high-quality services. Outcome measurement is also a requirement of the HCPC. Outcome measurement is core to:

- Delivering evidence-based and person-centred services.
- Evaluating clinical effectiveness and supporting quality improvement.
- Demonstrating the impact of speech and language therapy.

To support best practice in relation to outcome measurement, it is recommended that speech and language therapists are aware of the importance of:

- The routine measurement of the outcomes of therapy, using an appropriate approach and tools.
- The use of validated outcome measurement tools.
- Capturing the service-user's perspective on their outcomes and their experience of care.
- Using outcome data in the context of other data and alongside other available tools, frameworks and resources, to support the delivery of quality services.

Outcome measurement is embedded within a model of working that emphasises the need for reflection and holds the notion of health benefits and outcomes as an integral part of practice. As part of a programme of work on outcomes, the RCSLT has developed and piloted an online tool to support the collection of TOMs (Enderby and John, 2015, 2019). TOMs was selected as the 'best fit' tool after a systematic evaluation of available measures.

The RCSLT Online Outcome Tool (ROOT) supports speech and language therapists with the collection and collation of TOMs data and generating reports. The reports generated by the ROOT can be utilised by SLTs to inform clinical decision making and offer the potential to demonstrate the impact of SLT interventions for individual service users and cohorts of service users. In addition, the aggregated reports can be used to assist with service evaluation and quality assurances purposes, and to inform those funding speech and language therapy services.

SMART goals have been used for many years in different settings, with different opinions as to the author and originator of the process. SMART goals are based on the acronym:Specific, Measurable or Motivational, Attainable or Achievable, Realistic or Relevant and Time-based or Trackable. Goals are set according to those targets and in answer to questions of 'who, what, where, when, which and why' within each topic. They are, therefore, very much based on fact and are useful in demonstrating clinical effectiveness and involving the patient in joint goal setting at a level which the patient believes to be attainable. This encourages maximal participation and compliance.

The clinician's and patient's expectations in the outcome of therapy are very important, but must be based on the evidence and information available. It must not be directed by pressure from carers or through complaint, forcing compliance to provide a service, despite evidence that speech and language therapy is not the treatment of choice. It is certainly possible that change may occur in the patient's presenting symptoms, at which time reassessment may commence and new goals may be set.

Despite the wish that all patients would have an outcome of strong, normal voice, in reality this is not always possible. Clinicians should approach every patient with the knowledge that clinical effectiveness is not determined simply by whether the patient improves. Clinicians may provide the best quality of care for the patient using the most appropriate techniques of treatment, but find dissatisfying results because of factors outside their influence. It is best that this is discussed with the patient at the onset of therapy, with any potentially adverse factors noted by all involved. This enables appropriate clinical reasoning and decision making at the outset and assists in agreeing aims for the care episode. It is also imperative that these negative impact factors can be identified early so that both patient and clinician are aware of their influence on the potential outcomes of the therapy programme.

Prognostic indicators

In the clinical reasoning process and in considering the care plan for the therapy episode, the clinician may find it helpful to list predisposing, precipitating and perpetuating factors that will influence the outcome of therapy, in other words the prognostic indicators. This will help to form a realistic approach for the clinician which will be communicated to the patient throughout the therapy programme. A prognostic indicator checklist (Appendix VII) is included, offering an at a glance checklist of positive and negative factors to inform future treatment.

The laryngeal diagnosis and prognosis for recovery

The structure, appearance and function of the vocal folds in various disorders has been discussed fully previously, and has a great impact on the length of therapy and the potential outcome towards resolution of the disorder. This should be considered on the basis of the original laryngeal condition, its severity and its general prognosis, given all the best conditions for recovery. Many of the factors below will also influence laryngeal recovery, but will be considered separately.

Contributing factors

The case history should provide all the requisite information to allow an assessment of the patient's general health, hearing acuity, the environmental and occupational factors affecting their potential improvement and any personal factors such as bullying, harassment, burnout, stress and low morale, depression and disengagement, which could have a positive or negative impact on the outcome of therapeutic intervention.

The voice disorder

When a patient has a long-standing and untreated voice disorder, one could reasonably expect the entrenched patterns of voice use and vocal behaviour to be resistant to change. In the event of a recent disorder, the hope for a positive recovery should be increased given that the process of change is still in the early stages and may be positively altered. It may be appropriate to reiterate here that the evaluation of the patient according to the WHO

(ICF) categories of impairment, disability, handicap and well-being is helpful in the compilation of prognostic indicators.

Clinical decision making

There is much to be considered and there are many therapy approaches to the voice-disordered patient, from advice only to regular individual or group therapy options. Similarly, there should be an evaluation of the potential recovery and maintenance of normal voice, the probable timescale involved and the support likely to be given by friends, family and work colleagues.

Goal setting

Having chosen the most appropriate therapeutic programme, the clinician will begin to set goals for the patient that will dovetail exactly with the methodology used to demonstrate outcomes, as documented in the SOAP notes or the preferred method of documentation.

The following are some examples of how this might progress.

Specific targets for each session/short-term goals

The patient and clinician should have a clear sense of the goals of each session, having agreed the tasks at the beginning of the session, discussed them, experienced them through demonstration and self-practice, then reviewed them at the end. This might take the form of:

- using an agreed suite of relaxation exercises every day and completing a progress chart to evaluate the level of relaxation and ease with which this was achieved;
- targeting specific exercises for 10 minutes, twice per day for the next week, and trying to heighten awareness of the muscle movement and control involved;
- identifying and reducing irritants in the home and work environments;
- focusing on the reduction of specific elements of vocal misuse in a social setting through an agreed set of behavioural changes.

Week by week, these short-term goals work through the entire therapy programme, but with definite and current targets which keep the patient focused and realistic about the expectations of that week, while building towards the aims for the ensuing weeks.

Goals over several sessions/mid-term goals

Simultaneously there are general goals, which give stepping stones towards complete change and restoration of normal and adequate voice function, and which will last over several sessions or possibly the care episode:

- increasing awareness/applying relaxation of specific muscles in certain activities;
- improved posture and alignment during exercises and for specific activities;
- awareness of improved respiratory or vocal techniques during self-practice and specified situations;
- reducing/stopping smoking and reduction of irritants in the environment.

Outcomes of the care episode/long-term goals

Finally, there are the goals of achieving maximal change in all aspects of behaviour, resulting in reduction of contributing and perpetuating factors and establishing vocal adequacy for all situations. This will be demonstrated by whether the outcomes set at the beginning of the episode have been achieved, partially achieved or not achieved:

- optimal posture and balance of tension in all muscles at all times;
- awareness of potential stress and implementation of stress-reduction strategies in all situations;
- established vocal behaviour which is free from excess effort and adequate for all vocal loading;
- maximal change at home and work to facilitate an irritant-free environment.

As these three levels of targets are revised and reviewed regularly, there is clarity about what has been accomplished so far, the point reached in the patient's journey, and the ultimate aim of the intervention, all of which encourage motivation and perseverance to complete the process.

Options for therapy programmes

Length of the care episode

As mentioned earlier, the length of the care episode may vary greatly from one patient to another, between different commissioning authorities and indeed whether treatment is provided by the private or public sector. Whatever the likely length of the care episode, it is essential that the patient is aware of the number of sessions proposed and that the episode is not open-ended. The patient should also be aware that a subsequent care episode may be planned if necessary, but that the decision will be based on evaluation of the set goals and outcomes. Usually patients are pleased to have this information and can plan their time out of work or arrange personal commitments.

Length of therapy sessions

The clinician and the patient should agree the goal for each session. Similarly, they should both be aware of the planned outcome of the time together. In most authorities along with the initial therapy appointment the patient is sent an explanatory leaflet which is designed to help the patient understand what to expect from a Voice Therapy appointment, outlining the process of the first session, the length of the session, whether with a small group or on an individual basis and specific advice regarding any proposed assessment procedures. Ideally sessions should allow sufficient time for all planned therapy without any sense of haste, although of course this may have to alter as new information comes to the fore and requires discussion, or the patient may require more time than estimated to achieve the goal for the session. However, in all therapy, the clinician is the timekeeper who brings the sessions to a close at the appropriate time, hopefully having completed all that was planned. However, in practice, where there are high numbers of referrals, lengthy waiting lists and waiting times for therapy, there may well be some pressure on the time available and the clinician will have to adjust timing as appropriate, but the choices of therapy planning should allow sufficient flexibility for the unexpected.

Frequency of therapy sessions

Therapy sessions may be on an intensive daily basis, mentioned earlier in a 'Boot Camp' model as described by Patel *et al.* (2011). This may be necessary, for example, to accommodate a singer who is on tour for months at a time, for a patient who can only have therapy during a planned holiday, for someone who finds difficulty in retaining techniques from one session to another or where a psychogenic voice loss may be resolved within a few days of intensive therapy. As an episode of vocal rehabilitation, this plan gives little time for application of one block of the therapy programme before embarking on another, but if the patient fully understands the principle of building therapy block upon block, it is possible to have a successful outcome. Daily therapy, whether by daily physical attendance or on a virtual basis by telehealth, by its nature provides the blueprint of the required therapy aims and techniques, which should be achieved in the suggested order and timescale in the therapy plan. When a patient has made the commitment to 'attend' daily, one would hope for a good level of motivation to exercise consistently and apply the therapy plan over time.

These intensive treatment strategies require a high level of commitment from all involved and are obviously demanding in energy and time. The regularity of face-to-face treatment options are, as has already been said, entirely driven by the skills set and resources of the service and it is impossible to determine a country-wide pattern of intervention.

Individual or group therapy

Although individual therapy sessions may be the routine practice in many clinics, as noted earlier in this chapter, it can be valuable to consider group therapy for various reasons. Some patients find the anonymity of a group helpful in carrying out exercises, others feel supported and encouraged by the presence of others with similar difficulties. The group dynamic can be very positive in increasing motivation and the fulfilment of behavioural change, with group members often showing unexpected openness and receptivity to one another. It goes without saying that careful monitoring of the group is required to ensure that self-disclosure does not go beyond acceptable limits of advice and intrude on personal privacy and choice. For many voice patients, voice loss or alteration in vocal quality is a traumatic life event, affecting issues such as self-identity and future occupational choice. Pennebaker (1997) contends that the act of verbally encoding, by writing or speaking of traumatic life experiences, alters the way these events are stored in memory and can result in improved physical and mental health. Although support of Pennebaker's views is not universal (Kloss and Lisman, 2002), it is the experience of the author that group members will recount memories of helpful group activities and interaction many years after the end of a group programme.

Groups may fulfil different objectives, such as vocal rehabilitation, focus on a specific therapy intervention, initiate behavioural change, relaxation, stress reduction or include discussion on aspects of vocal usage. While clinicians may consider at length the composition of a group, there can also be surprises in the success of what may seem to be an ill-matched group of people. However, there are considerations for group work in terms of the number and experience of the clinicians available, the involvement of students or assistants, the number of patients to be involved, and the suitability of the facilities for the number of people attending at one time. Care should be taken to assess the demands of the group against the resources available, so that the duty of care is not compromised. Voice Information Groups have been mentioned in previous chapters as the first contact with the patient; an outline programme is provided in Chapter 7 and they will also be discussed more fully in Chapter 8.

Previous episodes of voice disorder

If this is a recurring disorder, there is a question over the causative factors in the recurrence and the responsibility taken by the patient either to seek or implement advice in previous episodes. However, ignoring a disorder should not always be thought to be due to a lack of motivation. Patients may live with a problem in the hope that it will eventually resolve spontaneously, due to fear of illness and hospital attendance, or as a result of irrational fear or phobia. Despite previous episodes of dysphonia, it should be clarified if this is truly a recurrence of the same problem or a different disorder. It is not uncommon for patients to progress well for years after a programme of voice therapy only to find that an illness or stressful event triggers a recurrence. It should not, therefore, be assumed that previous therapy has failed. Indeed, having completed a previous course of therapy the patient may be well motivated to comply and may make a speedy recovery. In the event that previous therapy has been unsuccessful, it is advised that the clinician attempts to gain the clinical notes from that episode or at least to determine from the patient their perception of lack of success. This may not be possible if the event was many years previous.

At first sight it may seem that the use of prognostic indicators is somewhat subjective, but it should be remembered that these indicators are based on much information from interview and assessment, as well as the sound clinical reasoning of the clinician. They are, however, only indicators and are not absolute judgements. They assimilate many facets of the data gained; they provide direction for the clinician in their patient management and treatment planning, and they may be changed as new details are discovered, with a subsequent revision of approach. In short, they provide another tool for the clinician in determining the best approach to management strategies and in planning aims for the short and long term.

Summary

In bringing together different aspects of clinical intervention and exploring the role they play, alongside strategic management choices, this chapter has focused on the importance of a number of diverse factors, from synergy between treatment efficacy and effectiveness, patient-centred care and patient-reported outcome measures to therapy outcome measures.

For that reason a wide range of issues from clinical skills, clinical roles, clinical effectiveness, clinical treatment programmes, therapy approaches, personal stress and prognostic indicators have all been considered.

The aim, as always, is to offer practical and experiential advice to support clinical practice while recognising that the clinician's focus is the provision of the best, most efficient and effective care episode possible for every patient.

THERAPEUTIC INTERVENTION

Introduction

In general, there is no one 'correct' set of exercises for a specific voice problem. Most voice problems, as has already been noted, comprise more than one feature and have more than one precipitating factor. The author is of the opinion that targeting discrete components of voice production is not particularly effective. A voice disorder is generally the result of a constellation of factors, so achieving change depends on a multifactored and nuanced approach. While different clinicians will select different approaches to achieve change, intervention strategies usually have a common denominator. Voice therapy, as was noted in Chapter 6, is an interaction between clinician and patient so it is possible that while one approach to a specific voice problem may work well for one clinician/patient dyad, for another a different approach will be better. Most (but not all) intervention begins by establishing effortless voice production in the clinic, followed by incremental challenges by way of length of continuous voicing, until fully integrated into conversational speech.

Treatment approaches

A range of treatment strategies are available to the clinician, from which a selection will be made depending on the clinician's assessment as to what best suits the particular patient's needs. These needs will encompass vocal rehabilitation, behavioural management, preference as to the style of exercises, available resources and attendance factors. Overall clinical judgement will dictate intervention.

In this chapter the emphasis is on practical exercises offering a firm foundation to establish an integrated physical and vocal approach to voice rehabilitation, an approach which, it is hoped, will be helpful both to the clinician and the patient, in that they target discrete areas of voice work from release of tension to resonance. There are exercises both for individual patients and for groups, such as occupational voice users (OVUs), in the shape of Teachers' Workshops. There is also a proforma outline for Voice Information Groups.

As with any discipline, the choice of intervention will depend on a number of issues, some of which will come down to the clinician's personal preferences, personal experience and indeed previous expertise. Clinicians will want to work within specific boundaries which are dictated by treatment approaches. Many clinicians will in fact use several different techniques at different times during intervention. Specific approaches or techniques of voice intervention are many and various, but it is important that in the adoption and use of a particular technique, the clinician continues to assess efficacy and outcome measures.

Therapeutic approaches are only as good as the clinician who is using them; as ever, the clinician holds the key.

An overview of several different approaches is outlined below, many of which may be familiar to readers. It is not in any way an all-inclusive list, nor is the inclusion or omission of certain approaches significant; neither is there any particular meaning to the order in which these are presented.

The Accent Method (Smith and Thyme, 1976; Thyme-Frøkjær and Frøkjær-Jensen, 2001; Stemple *et al.* 2013) is a holistic approach based on the principles of the myoelastic-aerodynamic theory of voice production. The Accent Method is designed to increase pulmonary output, improve glottic efficiency, reduce excessive muscular tension and normalise the vibratory pattern during phonation. The main goal of the Accent Method is 'to resolve pathological symptoms by optimising normal functions and to do this by achieving the best possible coordination between breathing, voicing, articulation, body movement and language for each individual' (Thyme-Frøkjær and Frøkjær-Jensen, 2001).

The approach has three major components – breathing exercises, phonatory exercises and movement exercises. This programme uses rhythmic exercises to facilitate the coordination of minimally constricted vocal fold vibration with appropriate air pressure and airflow. Rather than focusing separately on pitch, loudness and timbre, the Accent Method focuses on all three simultaneously. The Accent Method does not attempt to treat vocal pathology – its focus is on training patterns of voice production to encourage healthy conditions for voice and speech. Rhythmic contraction of the muscles involved in breathing is coordinated with production of increasingly complex utterances and the consonants in these utterances are used as accents within the rhythm. Initially, rhythmic whole-body movements are accompanied by rhythmic beating of a drum to facilitate clear and easy voice production. Rhythmic variation in pitch and loudness is incorporated to gain increased vocal flexibility. The graduated training exercises, modelled by the clinician and copied by the patient, move from simple to increasingly complex rhythms. Clinicians are strongly advised to attend a course on the Accent Method therapy to become familiar with the practice and theory of the method. In the UK the British Voice Association (BVA) delivers courses which set out the rationale on which the Accent Method is based, to allow delegates to experience the technique themselves and provide them with practical skills and tools to bring into their own area of work. The efficacy of the Accent Method of voice therapy is well established over many decades (Smith and Thyme, 1976; Kotby *et al.*, 1991; Fex *et al.*, 1994; Bassiouny, 1998; Malki *et al.*, 2008).

Estill Voice Training™ is a practical approach to voice work which relies on the individual gaining the ability to isolate and exercise independent control over certain parts of the vocal tract, for example, to raise and lower the larynx. These actions are known as 'Compulsory Figures' and are taught by trained practitioners who are licensed to train others. Specific figures are associated with a specific vocal quality, so titles such as 'sob', 'belting', 'twang' and 'opera' are readily identified by practitioners. Terms such as 'laryngeal tilt', 'anchoring' and 'desconstriction' are used to describe the independent movements. By acquiring the ability to consciously move each structure into two or three possible positions, the potential for controlled change of voice quality is increased. Synthesised into a creative system it offers an approach for therapeutic intervention as well as for professional voice users and singers. As with the Accent Method, the Estill Model is a system that is used throughout the world and practitioners need training to undertake the work. The Estill Voice training programme does not focus on breathing as a foundation for voice work but identifies the structures in the larynx responsible for producing voice and those in the vocal tract or throat responsible for controlling resonance and voice quality. Using sounds common to everyone, these structures are identified, isolated and then used to develop conscious, voluntary and predictable control of the voice.

Confidential Voice Therapy (Colton *et al.*, 2011) is an approach where the patient is encouraged to concentrate on making their voice as quiet and as breathy as possible, as though (as the name of the approach suggests) they are telling someone else a secret. The authors suggest that the use of breathy foundation has the added benefit of reducing loudness, rate and hyperfunction and heightens the awareness of allowing the expiratory airflow to do the work of producing sound. As it is a softly produced voice it is therefore not functional for many communicative needs, so confidential voice is designed to be used in acute (short-term) voice problems and after surgery to help facilitate mucosal repair. As part of a modified voice rest programme it can be used as the sole method of voice production for one to two weeks, or as part of a longer-term programme alternating periods of voice rest with more demanding voice use. Critical to the success of this approach is the low effort involved in phonation. However, low effort does not imply low pitch – importantly, normal pitch is maintained and a slightly sing-song pitch encouraged to prevent laryngeal inflexibility, which can prevent mucosal repair.

Resonant Voice Therapy has the goal of a more forward vocal placement. Patients are taught to feel the sensations of voice production in the palate, tongue and lips rather than in the throat. This approach focuses upon achieving a specific configuration of the vocal folds and muscles immediately above the vocal folds (the epilaryngeal area) by training the patient

The focus of the LMT technique is to decrease excessive contraction of the intrinsic and extrinsic muscles of the larynx. This is achieved through focal massage targeting selected areas of the vocal tract in a measured and incremental manner. It is carried out after palpatory evaluation of the perilaryngeal musculature and consists of rotational massage, kneading and stretching of those muscles. LMT is directed initially at the sternocleidomastoid muscles and subsequently at the supralaryngeal area. A full and detailed explanation of this technique is provided by Mathieson *et al.* (2009). The patient does not vocalise throughout the process of LMT until after the larynx responds easily to lateral digital pressure in the final stage of intervention.

MCT is achieved through pressing on selected areas of the neck (focal palpation) and manual repositioning of the larynx. Using the thumb and forefinger, moderate pressure is applied in small circles, from front to back, targeting selected areas of the larynx and neck. Laryngeal massage will therefore often focus initially upon the contracted thyrohyoid space (the area between the larynx and the hyoid bone) to release the excessive contraction and allow the larynx to descend. 'Gentle' (patients can express some discomfort during these procedures) manual repositioning of the larynx during phonation can sometimes prevent habituated patterns of excessive contraction. Unlike the process of LMT, vocal exercises are incorporated during the massage to facilitate clear and easy voice production without excessive muscle contraction and to allow the individual to hear resulting changes in voice quality (Andrews, 2006; Roy *et al.*, 1997).

Myofascial release is used to facilitate reduction and elimination of tension in the laryngeal muscles, as with Perilaryngeal Manual Therapies. It is used to address the tight muscles around the neck and hyoid, as well as the postural muscles that affect vocal quality and projection. Myofascial release is a hands-on technique that involves applying gentle, sustained pressure into the myofascial connective tissue targeted to release tissue restrictions in the neck, back, chest and abdominals. As with other perilaryngeal procedures, care, through properly designed protocols and/or training, needs to be taken by the clinician to avoid any adverse events, such as the patient experiencing light-headedness or dizziness due to carotid compression. Interventions should never be undertaken by novice providers without training. Training in MT techniques is the best way to avoid these events. Based on research and from clinical experience, myofascial release in combination with work with other professionals has shown to work well (Krisciunas *et al.*, 2019), thus supporting the findings of Marszalek *et al.* (2012) that the use of osteopathic myofascial therapy appears to significantly improve the functions of the vocal tract in patients with occupational dysphonia.

Semi-occluded vocal tract (SOVT) exercises in voice therapy involve narrowing at any supraglottic point along the vocal tract in order to maximise interaction between vocal fold vibration (sound production) and the vocal tract (the sound filter) and to produce resonant voice.

Straw phonation is one of the most frequently used methods to create semi-occlusion in the vocal tract (Titze, 2006, Titze and Verdolini Abbott, 2012). Narrowing the vocal tract increases air pressure above the vocal folds, keeping them slightly separated during phonation and reducing the force of the impact as they meet. To achieve this, the patient semi-occludes the vocal tract by phonating through a straw or tube. Through varying the length and diameter of the straw, resistance can be manipulated. Practice involves sustaining vowels, performing pitch glides, humming songs, and transitioning to the intonation and stress patterns of speech. The objective is to reduce the use of the straw and eventually eliminate it altogether.

Semi-occlusion at the level of the lips is accomplished via lip trills. This technique involves a smooth movement of air through the oral cavity and over the lips, causing a vibration (lip buzz), similar to blowing bubbles underwater. Often, the trills are paired with phonation and pitch changes. The focus is to improve breath support and produce voice without tension. When patients are working on SOVT exercises it is usual to have them sitting in an upright posture with shoulders in a low, relaxed position to facilitate voice production with less effort. Cielo *et al.* (2013) also found that the majority of studies show positive effects generated by SOVT exercises, such as improving proprioception and vocal self-control, the auditive-perceptive vocal aspects, the resonance subjects, projection and type of voice, acoustic vocal subjects such as reduction or increase of f0, reduced noise and increased harmonic energy, improve recordings' spectrogram, increasing the number of harmonics. Guzman *et al.* (2013) reported that researchers found that SOVT exercises may increase vocal economy by reducing phonation threshold pressure and effort while increasing or maintaining consistent acoustic output. Computerised tomography (CT) and acoustic results indicated that vocal exercises with increased vocal tract impedance lead to increased vocal efficiency and economy. One of the major changes was the more prominent singer's/speaker's formant cluster. Meerschman *et al.* (2019) investigated the effect of three SOVT therapy programmes: lip trill, water resistance therapy (WRT) and straw phonation on the vocal quality, vocal capacities, psychosocial impact and vocal tract discomfort of patients with dysphonia. Their results suggest that SOVT therapy programmes including lip trill or straw phonation can improve the objective vocal quality. Auditory–perceptual improvements (grade and roughness) were found after straw phonation therapy, whereas psychosocial improvements were found after lip trill and WRT. Patients seemed to experience more comfort and a better self-perceived vocal quality after WRT. Their study supports the use of the three SOVT therapy programmes in clinical practice: they all had a positive impact on one or more outcomes of the multidimensional voice assessment. What was most striking was the fact that vocal quality outcomes were not in line with the subject's opinion, so the authors recommend that a larger-scale investigation is needed to support their preliminary findings.

Cup bubble/Lax Vox technique, also known as Lax Vox, is an aerodynamic building task aimed at improving ability to sustain phonation while speaking. It is done by having a patient blow air initially into a cup of water without voice. Voicing can be added for subsequent trials and, in time, pitch can be altered across and within trials. Eventually, the cup is removed during voicing, and the phonation continues. These exercises are thought to widen the vocal tract during phonation and reduce tension in the vocal folds. Biofeedback increases the individual's awareness of his or her healthy voice production (e.g. Denizoglu and Sihvo, 2010; Simberg and Laine, 2007).

This book does not attempt to enlarge on these approaches, but advises reading and personal study, and attendance at specific training courses or conferences to learn in detail the techniques involved. While specific approaches may emphasise a particular philosophy and view of therapeutic intervention, they also encompass many features of conventional therapy which form the foundation for the voice to be rehabilitated and disorders resolved. These features or 'building blocks' of therapy are the emphasis of the rest of the chapter, providing a repertoire of treatment strategies; treatment strategies which will be effective in the remediation of the disorders described in previous chapters, as they lay strong foundations which can support subsequent vocal challenges. Without this 'building' model, there is always a danger of targeting an aspect of voice disorder in isolation and attempting inadequate and ineffective remediation or, indeed, causing an exacerbation of the disorder if, for example, the strong foundation for further work of posture and alignment, optimal muscle relaxation and adequate respiration is not included. However, the building model is also a holistic model, encompassing a 'whole-person', person-centred care approach to treatment planning.

Some of the exercises in this chapter may be familiar to readers in another form or from other sources. It is always difficult to correctly attribute provenance to exercises, but having worked with both Lyn Darnley and Myra Lockhart for many years, joint working, leading to a unity of approach and the development of a body of work, makes it almost impossible to attribute a specific practical exercise to a specific individual. The exercises in this chapter should therefore be considered as a joint endeavour and permission has been given to include them. It is very much hoped that none have inadvertently been appropriated without reference. The exercises included in this chapter offer a format which is patient-centred, easy to follow, and copies may be given to patients for home practise under the supervision of the clinician. It should also be recognised that the ordering of the exercises is not prescriptive, although it is suggested that posture, release of tension and breathing should be addressed in that order initially. Each of the exercise sections has an introductory practical advice page for patients, which, it is hoped, will provide a useful handout for patients and will underpin the graded exercises.

A number of Breathing and Voice workout exercises are included in this chapter which offer ideas for more maintenance-type intervention and may be used by patients once they have completed the more single-focus exercises. Two outlines for Teachers' Workshops are included; one is an example of content for a three-hour workshop and the other an example of content for a three-session format (Martin and Darnley, 2019). Also included is an outline of the content for a Voice Information Group. These have been used by the author and colleagues for many years and have therefore been 'stress tested' in various formats and settings and found to be effective.

For both the Teachers' Workshops and the Voice Information Group, it is advisable to include online resources of vocal fold movement. There are many online resources which give excellent images of the normal anatomy of breathing and voice, normal laryngeal and vocal fold movement and, in addition, images of vocal misuse and the impact on the larynx and the vocal folds. It is highly recommended that these are sourced and used in workshops, as most of those attending find them surprising and informative. The impact is often extremely high without being alarmist and increases motivation to change which is entirely self-generated by the patient.

Summary

The format for the exercises is that they should be practical and require no 'special' equipment of any sort. Each featured section begins with specific advice to be given to patients explaining the link between voice and the practical exercises. Clinicians will use their own judgement as to which exercises to use with which patient and also which exercises may be given to patients to work on at home without supervision. For various reasons, such as lack of space, some of the exercises may not be easily undertaken in the clinical setting, but will be helpful for the patient to try at home with prior guidance from the clinician. Some will be more suited to a specific patient; occupational voice users, for example, may well have different requirements to other voice patients. The choice, ultimately, is the clinician's.

POSTURE

Practical advice for patients

Making changes to habitual and long-held postural settings will take time and may initially feel uncomfortable as new 'muscle patterns' need to be established before becoming familiar.

The most effective standing posture involves a long spine in which the natural curves are maintained, with the head balanced in a relaxed and easy manner.

Poor posture affects the quality, volume and pitch of the voice, so when thinking about your posture the following advice may be helpful.

- If the spine is out of alignment, muscular stress will result, so keep your knee joints and thigh muscles relaxed when standing.

- Keep your pelvis level and try to balance your weight over both feet, with your feet 15–20 cm apart.

- Breathing and voice production are impaired if the ribcage is 'slumped' or constricted, so keep your ribcage relaxed and lifted to allow a virtual 'space' between the base of the ribcage and the abdominal area.

- Keep your shoulders in a neutral position, relaxed and lowered, counteracting any tendency to overcorrect or pull backward; this will decrease any tension in the upper chest area.

- If eye levels are too high or too low it will affect the positioning of the head and may lead to neck tension, so keep your head well balanced, with the crown of your head the highest point, so that it can move effortlessly in the horizontal and vertical planes.

- Poor neck alignment will create tension in the vocal tract, so by keeping your head level you will prevent a pull on the muscles of your neck and undue tension on your larynx.

- Good posture can also be achieved in the sitting as well as in the standing position.

Copyright material from Stephanie Martin (2021), *Working with Voice Disorders*, Routledge

POSTURE

Exercises to encourage good posture

A   Stand with your feet slightly apart and your weight evenly distributed

- Keep your knees relaxed, but flexible enough to allow forward and backward movement.

- Keep your pelvis balanced, not pushed too far forward or back.

- Raise first one arm and then the other, with the heel of your hand extended towards the ceiling.

- Now straighten your arms and gently punch the air above you with alternate hands.

- Note how this exercise frees the ribcage.

- Watch for any undue neck tension that can occur with this exercise unless carefully monitored.

B   Stand with your feet slightly apart and your weight evenly distributed

- Keep your knees relaxed, but flexible enough to allow forward and backward movement.

- Make sure that your pelvis is well balanced.

- Raise your arms above your head, but do not overextend them.

- Interlace your fingers with the backs of your hands pointing towards the ceiling.

- Maintain this position, but now reverse your hands so that, still interlaced, they are palm upwards to the ceiling.

- Now begin to 'walk' your hands towards the ceiling and feel the lift of the ribcage.

- Repeat this exercise three to four times.

- Note the increased space between your lower ribs and pelvis.

Copyright material from Stephanie Martin (2021), *Working with Voice Disorders*, Routledge

POSTURE

C Stand with your feet slightly apart and your weight evenly distributed

- Your knees should be relaxed but flexible.

- Raise your hands above your head and stretch towards the ceiling, but do not lift your heels off the floor.

- Maintain this stretch for about 30 seconds and then slowly start to lower your arms.

- Allow your head to follow this movement downwards, but do so in synchrony with the downward movement of your arms and shoulders. The weight of your head encourages the spinal column to curve.

- Fold over at the waist and bend at the knees, so that your arms swing freely.

- Hold this position and then gradually uncurl vertebra by vertebra until you are upright.

- Do not raise your head until you are completely upright.

- Monitor this new position and feel the reduction in any held tension.

NB: Do not attempt this exercise if you have problems with vertigo or dizziness.

D Stand comfortably with your weight well balanced and your head and spine in alignment

- Allow your shoulders, neck and back to relax.

- Breathe from your diaphragm and feel the movement in your lower chest.

- Remember to keep your shoulders and upper chest still but relaxed, not 'held'.

- Breathe out strongly as if sighing /hah/.

- Repeat this exercise two or three times.

- Now push your head forward and feel the tension.

- Note the pull on your larynx and neck muscles.

- Return to your former relaxed posture and try the exercise again, but this time add sound when you breathe out.

Copyright material from Stephanie Martin (2021), *Working with Voice Disorders*, Routledge

RELEASE OF TENSION

Practical advice for patients

Release of tension is important for efficient vocal function as breath support and control, volume, projection and vocal quality may all be affected by undue tension. It is quite possible to be relaxed when moving around freely, speaking and performing tasks, but it is important to remember that releasing tension is a technique like any other and it does need to be learned. While a degree of muscular tension is essential to support your body and to initiate and control movement, too much tension will affect smooth muscle coordination, which in turn will lead to general tiredness, strain and poor postural habits.

Do remember that habitual tension becomes 'normal' after a period of time and, because it is familiar, it does not seem out of the ordinary. It can be very difficult to identify the areas of the body that hold tension, so take time to develop an awareness of held tension before learning new techniques of tension release.

If you are feeling tense or wound up, your voice and speech will suffer, so when thinking about releasing tension the following advice may be helpful.

- Check on your tension levels throughout the day – be aware of any tension building up and try to counteract it. Allow enough time for exercises which release tension, and undertake these exercises in a space that is warm and comfortable.

- Listen to your own voice; make sure that the muscles in your throat and neck have not become tight.

- Encourage family, friends and work colleagues to help you to 'monitor' your tension levels.

- Try to make sure that you allow yourself some time each day for your exercises.

- Do not start your release of tension exercises in a hurry. Begin them when you are relaxed and quiet and do not rush them.

- If the time you have available for your release of tension exercises is limited, put them off until another time.

- Quiet background music is very helpful to aid the release of tension as you do the exercises.

Copyright material from Stephanie Martin (2021), *Working with Voice Disorders*, Routledge

RELEASE OF TENSION

- Limit any distractions before you begin the release of tension session, turn your mobile to silent, use the toilet, put a 'keep out!' sign on the door.

- Keep breathing slowly and steadily as you complete each exercise; do not breathe too deeply or too quickly.

- When you relax you need less oxygen and you breathe more slowly and more shallowly. Be aware of this happening as you relax.

Copyright material from Stephanie Martin (2021), *Working with Voice Disorders*, Routledge

RELEASE OF TENSION

Exercises to encourage general release of tension through imagery

A   Sit in a comfortable position with your eyes closed

- Think of a place which gives you a feeling of peace and relaxation. For example, this could be beside a warm fire or on a beach in the sunshine.

- Remember the feeling of warmth and peace that you experienced there.

- Add sounds to this image. Think of a favourite piece of music, or perhaps the sounds of the waves on the shore.

- Inwardly talk to yourself, using phrases such as, 'I feel calm and relaxed', or 'My tension is fading away'.

- Become aware of your breathing. Keep it slightly slower than normal and steady. Breathe in easily and breathe out in the same way.

- Enjoy the sensation of relaxation and be aware of how comfortable you feel.

B   Sit in a comfortable relaxed position with your eyes closed

- Think of somewhere quiet and peaceful. Use your memory as an aid.

- Use this image to encourage a feeling of peace.

- Keep this image of peace strongly in your mind.

- Slowly think through your body, from your toes to your head.

- Watch out for any areas of tension and release them muscle by muscle until your whole body is relaxed.

- Breathe in and out slowly, a little slower than normal but with no conscious effort at all.

Copyright material from Stephanie Martin (2021), *Working with Voice Disorders*, Routledge

RELEASE OF TENSION

Exercises to encourage progressive whole-body release of tension

A   Stand with your body well balanced

- Stretch your whole body upwards towards the ceiling, keeping your fingers extended.

- Feel the stretch in your spine and hold it for a few seconds.

- Start with the tips of your fingers, releasing the tension digit by digit.

- Allow your wrists to relax and flop, then your elbows, shoulders and head.

- Release tension through your spine, vertebra by vertebra, and allow your knees to 'give' a little.

- Allow your body to bob gently in this position.

- Reverse this sequence from the base of your spine, allowing each vertebra to build upon the preceding one.

- Finally, in a standing position, slowly raise your head and allow your arms to float weightlessly up to the starting position.

- You should experience a feeling of being light and stretched.

NB: Do not do this exercise if you suffer from vertigo or postural dizziness.

B   Sit comfortably in a firm chair with your back well supported by the back of the chair or lie down comfortably. If you feel any discomfort in your back, try lying with your knees raised a little, feet flat on the floor. Be careful not to press your feet into the floor, as this will create tension.

- Starting at your feet, curl your toes up as tightly as possible. Hold the tension for three to four seconds and then release it.

- Follow the same sequence of tensing, holding the tension briefly and then releasing while systematically working through your body, from the feet to the calves, to the knees to the thighs, buttocks, stomach, chest, back, hands, arms, shoulders, neck and, finally, the face and scalp.

Copyright material from Stephanie Martin (2021), *Working with Voice Disorders*, Routledge

RELEASE OF TENSION

- Remember that when you are thinking about your face you need to include the lips and tongue as well as the eyes and cheeks.

- Concentrate on achieving maximum tension each time, and then maximum release.

- Repeat each sequence of tension and release from tension three times with each muscle group.

- When you move from one muscle group to another, try to remember to maintain the release of tension in the muscles. Periodically revisit the areas and monitor any tension that may have returned.

- As you work through your body, concentrate on how it feels in a state of tension release. Your feet and hands should begin to feel slightly tingly, heavy and warm.

- Your legs should rest heavily into the chair if you are sitting, or on the floor if you are lying. Your stomach and waist should feel loose, soft and free, your arms resting heavily on the chair or on the floor, and at all times you should feel supported by the chair or the floor. You should not feel that you have to support your body in space unaided.

- As you work through your body from toes to scalp, become aware of your breathing. It should be slightly slower and steady. Feel the air as it flows in to fill your lungs and flows out as they empty.

- Sit or lie in this state of release from tension for a few minutes before moving, and then gradually bring yourself out of your state of released tension by thinking of moving and getting out of the chair or up from the floor. If you are moving from the floor, roll over on one side and then get up, making sure that you bring your head up last of all.

- Try and maintain this state of mind for as long as you can.

Copyright material from Stephanie Martin (2021), *Working with Voice Disorders*, Routledge

RELEASE OF TENSION

An exercise to encourage release of tension in the shoulders and upper chest

- Stand or sit comfortably in front of a mirror.

- Raise your shoulders as high as possible, straight up to your ears.

- Hold that position for a few seconds, then relax.

- Let your shoulders return to their resting position, gently sloping downwards.

- Repeat this several times.

- Become aware of the different muscle sensation between a state of tension and a state of release from tension.

Exercises to encourage release of tension in the neck muscles

NB: Any neck exercise must be done slowly and gradually and initially under the supervision of the clinician. Never force your neck.

A   You may sit or stand for this exercise

- With your head up and looking straight ahead, keep your eyes, nose and chin level.

- Slowly and gently turn your head to one side, until your chin is over your shoulder.

- Do not let your head tilt forward or back, be aware of where it is in relation to your body.

- Feel the stretch in the muscles of the side of your neck.

- Hold the stretch briefly, then slowly return to the midline.

- Repeat this sequence of movements to the other side.

- Repeat this three times on each side.

Copyright material from Stephanie Martin (2021), *Working with Voice Disorders*, Routledge

RELEASE OF TENSION

B Sit in a comfortable chair with your back well supported

- Drop your head slowly to one side towards one shoulder, feeling the muscle pull at the side of your neck.
- Now lift your head upright to the midline and repeat to the other side.

- Drop your head forward with your chin tucked to your chest and roll it to one side and then to the other.

- Now slowly lift your head and return to the midline.

- Repeat this sequence of movements three times.

Copyright material from Stephanie Martin (2021), *Working with Voice Disorders*, Routledge

RELEASE OF TENSION

An exercise to encourage a combination of whole-body release of tension with gentle voicing

- Sit in a chair in a relaxed position, with your feet on the floor and legs uncrossed.

- Make sure that your bottom is far enough back in the chair, so that your back is straight and supported by the chair.

- Check that your shoulders are level and not raised.

- Let your arms rest on the arms of the chair with your elbows low and touching the chair arms.

- Move your shoulders slightly, checking that they are not raised or tense. Use a gentle rotating movement to loosen them up before you start.

- Let your upper back, upper chest and ribs relax.

- Reach out with your right arm as if to take something, then let it rest back again in a relaxed position on the arm of the chair.

- Repeat the same action with your left arm.

- Allow your upper body to relax a little more.

- Slide your right foot forward slightly on the floor and then slide it back to a comfortable position with the leg relaxed. Do not exert any downward pressure as you do this.

- Now repeat the same action with your left foot.

- As you release tension, try to become aware of your breathing. When you release tension you need less oxygen and you breathe more slowly and more shallowly. Be aware of this happening as you relax.

- Feel how your diaphragm moves gently in and out as you breathe – you should feel its effect just above your waist. Do not force the breath in and out – allow this to happen naturally and spontaneously as you relax.

- Now try to breathe in slowly and a little more deeply and let the air come out again slowly, like a sigh. Breathe in through your nose and out through your mouth. Keep your

Copyright material from Stephanie Martin (2021), *Working with Voice Disorders*, Routledge

RELEASE OF TENSION

shoulders, neck, throat and jaw muscles free of tension so that you hear hardly any noise - just the sound of air through your relaxed throat.

- Now just breathe normally, but be aware of any tension and monitor this carefully.

- Making sure that you have remained free of tension, again take in a slightly deeper breath and slowly let the air out on a sigh. Release tension and breathe normally.

- Repeat this, but this time, instead of letting out a sigh, shape your lips into a rounded shape and let the air out on an /oo/ sound. Release tension and breathe normally.

- Breathe in and then out on an /ay/ sound. Release tension and breathe normally.

- Breathe in and then out on an /aw/ sound. Release tension and breathe normally.

- Now introduce a little voice when sighing out, so that the sound heard is /ha/. Release tension and breathe normally.

- Do the same but this time on /hoo/. Release tension and breathe normally.

- Then on /hay/. Release tension and breathe normally.

- Do the same with /hoh/. Release tension and breathe normally.

- Finish with /haw/. Release tension and breathe normally.

- Check that your breathing has remained slow and steady, and that your muscles have remained free from tension.

- Do not do this exercise too quickly. Leave plenty of time between each section to breathe normally several times, otherwise you could become light-headed.

Copyright material from Stephanie Martin (2021), *Working with Voice Disorders*, Routledge

BREATHING

Practical advice for patients

Breathing exercises can produce unexpected and uncomfortable emotional responses. This is quite a normal response and unless it brings back distressing memories or revives emotions that you cannot deal with there is no need to be concerned. The clinician will have seen the same response in other patients, so do not feel in any way embarrassed or uncomfortable. Do discuss any anxiety you feel with the clinician.

You may feel sceptical about needing to 'learn' to breathe, but in order to support your voice you need plenty of air and for that reason working on breathing and using your lower back and abdominal muscles is an important part of the breathing process. If you do not completely understand the explanation your clinician has given you regarding the connection between breathing and your voice, ask for more information.

When thinking about your breath, the following advice may be helpful.

- If your posture is a problem it is important to work on this before, or certainly alongside, work on breathing.

- Make sure that your lower back and abdominal muscles are not locked, as this will lead to tension and will limit the ease with which you can breathe.

- Use good, open posture and allow free movement of your whole body. Keep your back, shoulders and neck free from tension.

- Watch for any excess movement in your upper chest or shoulders. They should remain free from tension and still.

- Concentrating too much on breathing 'in' can cause tension in the upper chest and vocal tract, instead focus on the 'out' breath and the 'in' breath will follow more naturally.

- Silent breathing indicates relaxed, open air passages. Noisy inhalation and exhalation is caused by tension. If this occurs, try yawning widely to stretch and release the muscles in the throat.

Copyright material from Stephanie Martin (2021), *Working with Voice Disorders*, Routledge

BREATHING

- Be careful not to overbreathe. Only take two or three deep breaths at a time until your body becomes used to this new pattern, otherwise you may feel light-headed.

- If you suffer from asthma or respiratory problems, work within your own limits so that you feel secure and safe.

- Always remember to stop if you feel tired, light-headed, or short of breath. Release tension until the sensation has passed and always release tension between each attempt.

- Practising little and often is best.

Copyright material from Stephanie Martin (2021), *Working with Voice Disorders*, Routledge

BREATHING

Exercises to introduce diaphragmatic breathing

A Stand in front of a long mirror and place your hands on either side of your waist, with fingers spread and pointing towards the centre of your waist, thumbs behind and pointed towards the back

- Press firmly with your hands, as though trying to make them meet in the middle, and breathe out.

- Maintain your hand position and take a breath in, feeling the forward and side expansion.

- Watch in the mirror as the gap between your fingertips increases.

- Monitor your shoulder movement at the same time – there should be no undue movement.

B Stand in front of a long mirror. Place one hand on your midriff and exert some slight inward pressure

- Breathe in and monitor the outward movement of your midriff. Maintain a tension-free posture with no undue movement in your shoulders or upper chest.

- Breathe out on a /f/ sound. Feel your hand move inwards. Release tension and breathe normally.

- Repeat this several times.

- Remember that your hand moves out as the breath moves in.

Copyright material from Stephanie Martin (2021), *Working with Voice Disorders*, Routledge

BREATHING

C   Start with your feet slightly apart, and arms out to the sides

- On an outgoing breath, drop your arms. Then sweep them back up, with your palms uppermost. When they are at eye level in front of your body, allow your knees to bend.

- Drop your arms and sweep them back into their original position as you breathe in.

- Notice how the breath flows back into your chest.

- Return your arms to their forward position on the exhaled breath.

- Repeat for a maximum of 20 swings, or as many as are comfortable, always releasing tension and breathing normally between each attempt.

Copyright material from Stephanie Martin (2021), *Working with Voice Disorders*, Routledge

BREATHING

An advanced breathing exercise

Breathe out and eliminate as much air as possible from the lungs

- Feel the action in the centre of your body, but do not shorten your spine.

- Wait for a second or two.

- On the 'in' breath experience the sudden, dramatic and powerful inflow of air.

- Repeat this 5-10 times.

- Stop if you feel at all dizzy or unwell.

Copyright material from Stephanie Martin (2021), *Working with Voice Disorders*, Routledge

BREATHING

Exercises to encourage greater awareness of breath in the lumbar area

A   Lie face down with a heavy book placed on your lower back

- Breathe in and think about the breath low down in the lungs.

- Be aware of the book rising and falling as you breathe in and out.

- Remember this is due to the activity of the muscles which support breathing.

B   Sit back to front astride an upright chair

- Allow your spine to curve.

- Lean forward and place your arms on the back support.

- On the 'in' breath think about breathing low into the back area.

- Feel the sideways spread of your back.

- You may want to ask someone to put their hands on your lower back to help you feel this sideways movement more easily.

Copyright material from Stephanie Martin (2021), *Working with Voice Disorders*, Routledge

BREATHING

Exercises to encourage breath control

A Breathe in through your nose and out through your mouth, gently and easily, until a smooth and relaxed rhythm has been established

- Once you have achieved this, begin a silent count, breathing in for three seconds and breathing out for three seconds.

- Maintain this silent count for several attempts and then begin to vary the length of the 'in' and 'out' breaths.

- Try a count of two for the 'in' breath and four for the 'out' breath.

- If you find it difficult to maintain the silent count while concentrating on the breath pattern, then ask someone to count aloud for you.

- As you get better, decrease the 'in' breath time and increase the 'out' breath time. This more closely mirrors the pattern of breathing for sustained and controlled phonation.

- Breathe in on a count of two and out on the sound /s/ for as long as possible but without strain.

- Make sure that you do not allow any tension to occur in your lips, tongue or neck.

- If you do feel any tension occurring, reduce the length of time over which you maintain the /s/ sound.

Copyright material from Stephanie Martin (2021), *Working with Voice Disorders*, Routledge

BREATHING

B Sit in a position that is tension-free with your back supported and as upright as possible

- Relax your shoulders.

- Rest your arms on the arms of the chair or by your side, but ensure that they are not held tightly against your ribcage.

- Breathe in a tension-free and even pattern, with small amounts of air only.

- Breathe in slowly for three seconds, expanding the bottom of the ribcage and feeling the diaphragmatic movement. Pause briefly, then breathe out slowly for three seconds.

- Return to even, shallow breathing and release tension.

- Repeat this exercise four times, always breathing in for three seconds, pausing, breathing out for three seconds, then returning to natural breathing at rest.

Copyright material from Stephanie Martin (2021), *Working with Voice Disorders*, Routledge

BREATHING

Exercises to encourage control of breath pressure

A   Use different images to experiment with breath pressure, fitting the breath to the task

- Imagine blowing a feather off your hand.

- Imagine blowing out four candles on a cake.

- Imagine blowing out six everlasting candles on a cake.

- Imagine blowing to keep a balloon airborne for as long as possible.

- Imagine using breath to paint a picture where each colour is a different breath pressure.

- Never force the breath out or allow undue tension to affect the exercise.

B   Take in a moderate amount of air on an inward count of two and when you breathe out try to produce a long steady /ssssss/

- Do not produce the sound with any excess tension in your lips, tongue or neck. Do not force the air out, simply maintain a steady pressure and listen to the sound.

- As you become more competent you will find that you can maintain the /s/ sound for longer without undue effort.

- Begin to vary the loudness of the sound – make it quiet to begin with and then let it get louder – ssssSSSSSS.

- Begin with a loud /S/ sound but not forcefully and let it become quieter over time – SSSSssss.

- Vary the loudness so that the sound is loudest in the middle – ssssSSSSSssss.

- Try to alternate periods of loudness and quietness – sSsSsSsSsS.

- Try using /f/ or /sh/ in place of /s/ for these exercises, although you will need a little more air pressure to maintain these sounds as they may not last as long.

- Always aim for quality of sound, do not compromise quality for quantity.

Copyright material from Stephanie Martin (2021), *Working with Voice Disorders*, Routledge

BREATHING

C   Take in a manageable amount of air, but try not to over-breathe

- Make sure that you do not 'control' the sound by constricting your larynx, but control it from your diaphragm.

- Try to produce both a long /s/ sound (S) or a short /s/ sound (s), for example, SSSSsssSSSS or SsSsSs. Experiment on a variety of rhythms.

Copyright material from Stephanie Martin (2021), *Working with Voice Disorders*, Routledge

VOICE

Practical advice for patients

For most people, voice is something that just happens; you think of something to say, you say it, and how it happens is rarely, if ever, thought about. For voice patients, however, something has 'gone wrong' in that process and the voice no longer just 'happens'. It is particularly important that you know why your voice is not functioning as well as it should, so you are aware of what changes you need to make to keep it working and in good health.

If you feel very tense and anxious, ask the clinician for help with work on posture, release of tension and breathing before working on your voice.

Making changes to the way in which you use your voice requires careful attention and consistent effort, so when thinking about your voice the following advice may be helpful.

- Remember it is important to be gentle with your vocal folds; they will work very well if they are not ill-treated.

- Excess tension in the internal musculature of the vocal folds will stop them moving together smoothly and increase the load on the vocal folds.

- Monitor any excess tension in your chest and shoulders.

- Keep your neck and jaw relaxed.

- Make sure that you have enough air to support your voice before you start to speak.

- Think carefully about how you are coordinating your breath with your voice.

- Try not to 'punch' or 'force' the sound out.

- Ask the clinician to demonstrate any terms that you do not completely understand, for example, how to differentiate between hard attack and normal glottal closure.

- During the production of an /h/ sound the vocal folds do not fully close together, which reduces hard attack. Using an /h/ before a vowel sound will help you to do this and the clinician can give you exercises for this.

Copyright material from Stephanie Martin (2021), *Working with Voice Disorders*, Routledge

VOICE

Exercises to release tension and constriction of the vocal folds and the surrounding muscles

Use the following natural movements to help release tension and constriction. Some may feel more comfortable than others and allow you to feel the release of constriction. Use the ones which help best. If your muscles are very tense, the exercise may be slightly uncomfortable at first as you stretch and/or release this tension. Be gentle and gradually the tension will reduce.

- Breathe in as if you are smelling a beautiful perfume, aftershave or flowers. Breathe in deeply and feel your throat release constriction as you do this. Release tension and breathe normally. Repeat this several times with normal breaths in between.

- Imagine you have been given a wonderful surprise and you express your amazement by opening your mouth wide as if saying /aah/ while breathing in.

- Remember the feeling of coming home after a long, tiring day. As you settle into your favourite chair and kick off your shoes, you take in a deep breath and sigh a long and loud sigh. Your voice begins high and slides to a lower pitch as you sigh.

- Breathe in, then yawn widely and loudly. Feel the release of tension and constriction as you yawn.

- Holding an imaginary glass or large mug, tip the contents slowly over the back of the tongue and down the throat, feel the additional space that has been created.

- The Yoga Lion: suddenly (and simultaneously) stretch fingers with eyes wide open while stretching the tongue out of the mouth. Hold the position briefly and then gently release; the jaw and tongue will slowly return to their natural positions where they remain free of tension and neutral. Experience the space inside the mouth and the back of the throat.

- Place one hand in the centre of the body over the diaphragm and breathe out silently onto an imaginary mirror held in your other hand as if you were misting up the mirror. Make sure that the breath enters and leaves the body silently.

Copyright material from Stephanie Martin (2021), *Working with Voice Disorders*, Routledge

VOICE

Exercises to reduce tension in the vocal folds

A Breathe in using your diaphragm and without any shoulder or upper chest tension

- As you breathe out make a strong SSS sound, gradually increasing the loudness and flow of air.

- Repeat the same sequence, but this time, as the air flow increases, change the /s/ to a /z/ sound so that you hear, for example, sssssszzzzz with no break between the sounds.

- Repeat the exercise several times, aiming at a smooth change from /s/ to /z/.

- This shift from /s/ to/z/ encourages the vocal folds to vibrate in a tension-free manner to produce the voiced sound /z/.

B Try to combine your improved breath control with gentle voicing by saying sss...zzz...sss...zzz

- Gradually increase the length of this by alternating between /s/ and /z/ as many times as possible – sss...zzz...ssss...zzzz...sssss...zzzzz.

- Monitor any undue tension that might occur.

C Begin by taking in a moderate breath. Remember to monitor any tension in your shoulders, upper chest or back

- Use a strong flow of air from your lungs to achieve the first sound in the following non-sense words, and sustain this to lead seamlessly into the vowel. Use a falling pitch on the vowel as this helps to reduce tension:

sah	say	soo	sow	see
saw	so	sigh	soy	sar

Copyright material from Stephanie Martin (2021), *Working with Voice Disorders*, Routledge

VOICE

D As you become more confident, try the following short sentences, monitoring for tension and taking care not to 'push' to sustain voice - instead take another breath in the middle of the phrase if necessary

Sometimes she sends it.	Show me the same one.
Sam was always the same.	Sylvia started the song.
Should I shorten this or not?	Suppose I shop around?
Shopping centres are so busy.	She said it was simple to see.

Copyright material from Stephanie Martin (2021), *Working with Voice Disorders*, Routledge

VOICE

Exercises to reduce tension in the ventricular fold muscles

The muscles above the vocal folds are called the ventricular folds. When these muscles become very tense and work with too much effort a rather hoarse and rough vocal quality can result.

The following exercises transfer tension and effort away from these muscles and help to produce a clearer voice quality. They should never be used in isolation, but always in tandem with breathing and relaxation exercises.

A   Breathe in and out with relaxed back, chest and shoulders

- Next, take in a moderate amount of air and 'whistle' on the 'out' breath, but without undue effort and with rounded lips.

- Repeat this, noting the length of time that you can sustain the whistle.

- Gradually try to increase the length of time during which you can sustain the whistle.

- Keep a note of how many seconds you can achieve, and monitor your progress.

B   Breathe in and out, keeping a relaxed back, chest and shoulders

- Take in a moderate amount of air and with rounded lips say the word 'who' on the 'out' breath, trying to prolong the /oo/ sound.

- Make sure that you start to say the word as soon as you start to breathe out.

- Try not to let any air escape at the beginning without being used, as this reduces the control.

- Try to gradually increase the length of time that you can sustain the /oo/ for.

Copyright material from Stephanie Martin (2021), *Working with Voice Disorders*, Routledge

VOICE

C As you become more confident and can maintain the sound for longer without tension, try to produce a longer word with the same relaxed and clear voice

- Try the following words with rounded lips:

Whoever	Hoovering	Whooping

- Now try these slightly longer phrases:

Whoever it is	Hoovering up	Whooping it up

D As you become more able to achieve a clear and tension-free vocal note on short sentences, try the following longer ones. Remember to keep an overly rounded lip position for the first sound

Who is on the phone?	Who will be coming today?
Who called you?	You need to remember the number.
Use the right hand to open it.	When will you be able to tell me?
Which one is the best one?	Whatever you want is available.
Where will he be living in Spain?	We will always provide the best service.

Copyright material from Stephanie Martin (2021), *Working with Voice Disorders*, Routledge

VOICE

Exercises to encourage gentle closure of the vocal folds

A   Remember to release tension from your back, chest and shoulders. Try to maintain this sense of freedom from tension as you complete this exercise

- Breathe in, then breathe out a sigh /h/.

- Breathe in, then breathe out on a soft /hah/.

- Breathe in, then out on a soft /hoh/.

- Breathe in, then out on a soft /hey/.

- Breathe in, then out on a soft /hoo/.

- Breathe in, then out on a soft /hi/.

- Listen carefully as you are doing this exercise, in case any tension occurs.

- Repeat the same exercise, but this time put /sh/ not /h/ at the beginning of the word.

- Now try the same exercise with /f/ at the beginning of the word.

B   Try the following nonsense words, allowing yourself plenty of breath to support the voice

- Breathe in, and then out on /fu hu/.

- Breathe in, and then out on /su shi/.

- Breathe in, and then out on /fey how/.

- Breathe in, and then out on /fah say/.

Copyright material from Stephanie Martin (2021), *Working with Voice Disorders*, Routledge

VOICE

C   This time try some slightly longer nonsense words

- Breathe in, and then out on /foo soh shi/.

- Breathe in, and then out on /hoh sho fah/.

- Breathe in, and then out on /fee sha hi/.

- Now try some slightly longer words with four syllables.

- Breathe in, and then out on /say hoo fah si/.

- Breathe in, and then out on /fah say di hey/.

- Breathe in, and then out on /hay foh shi shu/.

- Always remember that it is the quality of sound that is important.

Think about making each sound clear but not forced, and remember it is important not to hear any hard attack at the beginning of the sound.

Copyright material from Stephanie Martin (2021), *Working with Voice Disorders*, Routledge

VOICE

D **Use this list of words to practise soft attack, but always remember to breathe before you start and try just one word at a time, breathing normally in between**

hoe	who	him	his	hill	high
his	home	house	ham	hat	hit
hen	hand	hound	hop	herd	hoard
hip	hum	harm	head	hail	hell
hem	half	hard	hope	hang	hue
say	see	sew	sigh	sue	sing
sill	sin	sand	sung	sell	sit
sound	suit	soup	sum	seed	soap
sip	same	sail	sat	surf	soar
fill	fed	fat	fell	fun	fan
fast	foil	foot	fit	file	fox
food	feel	fin	fuss	fee	fail
fax	fix	fate	feet	fish	far
shoe	shy	show	shop	she	shock
ship	sham	sheep	shale	shine	shape
share	shell	shore	sharp	sheriff	shirt
when	why	where	what	whale	whine
while	whisk	whom	whip	wheel	west
weight	what	wasp	wax	warm	wail
watch	want	wit	wipe	walk	wick
wood	wall	wife	wad	will	well

Copyright material from Stephanie Martin (2021), *Working with Voice Disorders*, Routledge

VOICE

E **With this exercise it is important to listen to the contrast between those words that begin with /h /and those that begin with a vowel. Try to allow a little puff of air to come through your vocal folds before you say the words beginning with the vowels**

hoe	oh	ham	am
high	eye	harm	arm
heat	eat	hair	air
hill	ill	hand	and
his	is	handy	Andy
hat	at	hark	ark
hear	ear	hedge	edge

F **Use the short puff of air to lead into these phrases**

I might
all over
air waves
alterations off
every one
even then
except this one
after all is over
I am all ears
I always go out then
I always go out at eight
I am trying to connect you
I am having some difficulty
It's outside on the grass
It might take some time

- Try to let one word flow into the next, so that there is no sharp break between words.

- Keep the air flowing strongly and with control through to the end.

- Become aware of this new way of using your voice.

- Begin to practise on phrases that you use often at home or at work and which begin with vowels.

Copyright material from Stephanie Martin (2021), *Working with Voice Disorders*, Routledge

PITCH

Practical advice for patients

If you have been concerned about the pitch of your voice, changing to one that seems to better 'fit' your age and gender may well feel uncomfortable initially. Family, friends and colleagues may take some time to 'accept'/'get used to' the new pitch and indeed may well comment on it. Discuss how you are going to deal with questions or comments with your clinician. You may want to apply your new pitch gradually or only in certain situations initially.

Most importantly, do not force your voice, do not try to speak at a higher or lower pitch until you have completed the exercises in clinic, and if you feel any discomfort using your new pitch, stop and discuss this with your clinician.

In working on altering the pitch of your voice the following advice may be helpful.

- Any general tension should be eliminated before working on pitch, as tension will limit your vocal range and flexibility by inhibiting the vertical movement of the larynx and the smooth approximation (coming together) of the vocal folds.

- If you find it difficult to achieve alteration to your pitch, feel the vertical movement of the larynx during pitch changes. If that does not help, digital manipulation of the larynx by the clinician may be a useful way into work on pitch.

- Once you have achieved the new pitch, work on consolidating it, so it becomes habitual.

- Try to carefully monitor the new pitch by listening attentively as you use your voice and noting any periods where your voice returns to the pre-therapy pitch.

- Encourage flexibility and range within the pitch by allowing the vocal pitch to respond naturally to changes in thought and emotion.

Copyright material from Stephanie Martin (2021), *Working with Voice Disorders*, Routledge

PITCH

Exercises to encourage variety of pitch

A   The following contrasting pairs of words can be used to encourage you to use high and then low pitch alternately

High pitch	Low pitch
ping	pong
ding	dong
high	low
hill	valley
sky	sea
excited	bored
soft	hard
treble	bass

- Try to add to the list with words that you associate with high or low pitch.

B   The meaning of some words seems to encourage a high or low pitch

- Try the following words with the appropriate pitch:

High pitch				
screech	creak	cheep	shrill	tiny
squeak	piercing	whistle	cry	yelp
sing	giggle	spring	twinkle	trill
Low pitch				
dark	malice	grumble	grim	sink
growl	grave	doom	snore	dank
glower	shudder	dive	moan	growl

- Try to add to this list yourself.

Copyright material from Stephanie Martin (2021), *Working with Voice Disorders*, Routledge

PITCH

C As you use your voice in conversation, think about the pitch you use and also note the variety of pitch changes that other people use

• Try to combine high and low pitch in words and sentences.

• Start with the months of the year and say the months with alternate high and low pitch.

D A similar exercise can be done with a series of numbers

• Try the following series of numbers, rising in pitch with each number:

123	211	569
678	679	237

• Try slightly longer numbers:

123467	532124	8510067

• Now try the same series of numbers, but start with a high pitch and lower it.

E Once you can achieve a gradual rise in pitch, try to do the same with short sentences

I can climb higher and higher.

The balloon flew higher and higher in the sky.

The kite rose so high it was soon out of sight.

• As an alternative, try to start with a high pitch and gradually lower it:

The ice-cream melted and fell on the ground.

The sun dropped lower and lower in the sky.

The rocket nose-dived into the sea.

F Exercises to encourage flexibility of pitch

• Read a children's story as though to a small child.

• Use an exaggerated up-and-down pitch pattern.

• Go through a short paragraph in a newspaper underlining every verb. Read the paragraph aloud, and on every underlined word allow for an extreme rise in pitch.

Copyright material from Stephanie Martin (2021), *Working with Voice Disorders*, Routledge

MUSCULAR FLEXIBILITY

Practical advice for patients

Making changes to articulatory movements may feel uncomfortable and strange initially and can indeed seem exaggerated and unacceptable.

As with work on breathing exercises, work on the jaw, lips and tongue can produce unexpected and uncomfortable emotional responses. This is quite a normal response as emotional tension can be held in these areas. For example, one hears, 'keep a stiff upper lip', grit your teeth', 'bite your lip to stop crying'. Unless the work brings back distressing memories or revives emotions that you cannot deal with there is no need to be concerned. Do discuss any anxiety you feel with the clinician.

If you feel that work on your jaw, lips and tongue does not fully take into account cultural considerations, this should be discussed with the clinician. In certain languages, for example, only a moderate amount of jaw opening is used when speaking; in certain cultures female speakers protect the lower half of their face in public and so may feel uncomfortable with exaggerated facial movement.

Lack of muscular flexibility affects the effective and efficient use of the voice. Speech which is imprecise and difficult to understand will detract from the communicative process, resulting in a loss of meaning, so for that reason it is essential that the lips, tongue soft palate and pharynx are as mobile as possible, so when thinking about muscular flexibility the following advice may be helpful.

- Tension causes muscular inflexibility, so before beginning any work on increasing muscular flexibility, start with a yawn and a stretch, which not only releases tension but also stimulates energy.

- Muscular flexibility exercises should be done at a moderate speed initially. Do not try to rush through the exercises – speed is not a criterion of success. Precision is more important than speed.

- Make sure you are not holding your breath when completing the exercises.

Copyright material from Stephanie Martin (2021), *Working with Voice Disorders*, Routledge

MUSCULAR FLEXIBILITY

- When working on muscular flexibility, always use a mirror to give you visual and kinaesthetic feedback.

- Try to think of each movement separately, and build up the sequence gradually.

- If you are in a young/youngish age group, where limited muscularity is often the norm, recognise that peer pressure and comment may be an issue.

- Use your 'new', more precise articulation when talking on your mobile/landline phone initially, until you feel more comfortable with what may appear (to you) to look like a very over-exaggerated way of speaking.

NB: It is always important to be aware that poor flexibility can be the result of neurological impairment and, if so, practice will not make perfect. If you are in any way concerned about your ability to carry out the exercises do not hesitate to discuss this with your clinician, although this is a topic that will have been addressed when your case history was taken.

Copyright material from Stephanie Martin (2021), *Working with Voice Disorders*, Routledge

MUSCULAR FLEXIBILITY

Exercises for the jaw

Remember to keep the tongue relaxed when doing these exercises.

A Clench your teeth together tightly

- Now release the tension that is keeping the teeth together and feel the difference.

- Try this several times, but do not overdo this exercise.

- Remember how the clenched jaw feels and use this to monitor your jaw position periodically throughout the day.

- Release any undue tension.

B Place your fingers on either side of your face at the level of the jaw

- Stroke the jaw downwards, allowing it to open gently, little by little.

- Keep your lips in light contact at all times.

- Feel the separation of your upper and lower teeth.

C Keep your lips lightly together

- Chew an imaginary piece of toffee quite vigorously for a while.

- Monitor the tension level.

- You may notice some slight discomfort in the jaw initially – this is because the movement is unaccustomed and more vigorous than you are used to.

- This will disappear with practice, but do mention it to your clinician if you are concerned.

Copyright material from Stephanie Martin (2021), *Working with Voice Disorders*, Routledge

MUSCULAR FLEXIBILITY

Exercises to encourage an open pharynx

A   Imagine you are chewing a piece of toffee, which becomes bigger as you chew

- Make the movements of your jaw more vigorous, and open your mouth to accommodate the increasing size of the toffee.

- With jaw exercises, be aware of but not worried about any discomfort, unless it is particularly bad.

- Notice that your pharynx is more open on completion of this exercise.

B   With a relaxed, open jaw, push your tongue as far out of your mouth as possible

- Now try to say a nursery rhyme with your tongue still out.

- With your tongue back 'in place' say the nursery rhyme again and be aware of the difference in quality and the feeling of space in your pharynx.

C   Relax your lips and try to smile 'inside' your mouth

- Be aware of the feeling of space and openness in your pharynx.

D   Keep your lips together with very light contact

- Try to produce a full yawn.

- Be aware of the feeling of space and openness in your pharynx.

Copyright material from Stephanie Martin (2021), *Working with Voice Disorders*, Routledge

MUSCULAR FLEXIBILITY

Exercises to encourage lip mobility

A   Purse your lips, maintaining quite firm contact

- Rotate them in a clockwise direction and repeat several times.

- Stop and release contact before beginning the exercise again in an anti-clockwise direction.

- Repeat this exercise several times.

- Once you are confident, try to change direction frequently without stopping.

B   Blow out air through your lips so that they vibrate rapidly

Feel the movement in your lips and be aware of the residual tingling.

C   Press your lips together

- Keeping the air pressure within your mouth, blow out your cheeks.

- When you have done this, lightly tap your fingers against your cheeks and release the air with a 'pop'.

D   Curl your upper lip up towards your nose

- Try to balance a pencil on your lip.

- Remove the pencil.

- Try to curl your lower lip down towards your chin.

Copyright material from Stephanie Martin (2021), *Working with Voice Disorders*, Routledge

MUSCULAR FLEXIBILITY

Exercises for the tongue

A   Stick your tongue out of your mouth

- Make the tip into a thin, pointed shape.

- Now spread the sides of the tongue so they become wider and flatter.

- Keep alternating these positions.

B   Stick your tongue out of your mouth with the tongue-tip pointed

- Use it like a pen to 'draw' a picture.

- Now try to 'write' the title of a book or a film.

C   Tuck the tip of your tongue behind your lower front teeth

- Flatten the rest of your tongue, but keep it in your mouth.

- Now bunch your tongue forward and try to push it out of your mouth.

- Remember to keep the tip of your tongue behind your lower front teeth.

Copyright material from Stephanie Martin (2021), *Working with Voice Disorders*, Routledge

MUSCULAR FLEXIBILITY

Exercises to encourage increased precision in the use of the articulators

A   Both lips

A big beetle blithely bit a big black box of beans.

Many merry moments made the millennium memorable.

A pale purple peahen perched perilously on the parapet.

Melon, mushroom, marmalade and mackerel were munched by the monkey.

B   Tongue tip and alveolar ridge

A dozen double damask dinner napkins.

A single solid silver sifter sifts sifted sugar.

A rural ruler recognised rural rivalry and resolved to rally the unruly ruffians.

A roving raven relinquished the wretched rabbit.

C   Lower lip and upper teeth

Five French firemen fanned a fainting friar.

Four flippers flashed as two frisky dolphins swam fast and fleetingly.

Phyllis found a fancy fan finely fixed with three fluffy feathers.

D   Tongue tip and upper teeth

Three thousand thin thrushes thrilled them.

The sixth sick sheikh's sixth sick sheep.

The Leith police dismisseth us.

Copyright material from Stephanie Martin (2021), *Working with Voice Disorders*, Routledge

MUSCULAR FLEXIBILITY

E Tongue blade and front of hard palate

Cheerful children chanting charming tunes to cheer Charles.

Joan joined John in jumping Jack's jolly jam jar.

If a dog chews shoes what shoes does she choose to chew?

F Back of tongue and soft palate

A cup of creamy custard cooked for Christmas.

The coal in the school coal scuttle was scattered by a cold scholar.

Occupying an old oak the old owl ogled the odious ostrich.

For the professional voice user it is particularly important that sounds are not substituted, for example, a /ch/ is often used instead of a /t/ in the following words: tune, tutor, tube, tuna, Tuesday. Equally, some sounds are elided or final consonants lack clarity.

Copyright material from Stephanie Martin (2021), *Working with Voice Disorders*, Routledge

RESONANCE

Practical advice for patients

Making changes to the resonance or overall tonal quality of your voice will take time as it can be difficult to fully identify different resonant qualities in your own voice. There are three principal resonators of the voice: the pharyngeal, the oral and the nasal resonators. Limited oral resonance can make your voice sound 'thin' and too little nasal resonance can make it sound as though you have a cold.

Listening to your voice and identifying the different resonators is something you will have been working on with the clinician. It is important to increase your auditory awareness and understand the way in which the different resonators affect your vocal quality. When thinking about resonance, the following advice may be helpful.

- Keep free from tension and think about your posture and how you are using your breath to support the sound when you are trying the exercises.

- Be aware of any residual tension or constriction you may be holding in the vocal tract as that will affect resonance.

- Try to make sure your tongue, jaw, neck and larynx are free from tension before attempting the exercises.

- The quality of the laryngeal note is of critical importance when working on resonance.

- Some regional accents make greater use of nasal resonance than others and it is generally accepted that American English is more nasally resonated than British English. Your exposure to different cultures and languages will influence you when initiating change.

- Resonance can be confused with volume or pitch level, so discuss this with the clinician so you know exactly what you are working on.

- Working on resonance will give your voice a full, rounded sound rather than a thin one.

- Listen to the different resonance of different speakers in order to familiarise yourself with the difference that certain resonators bring to vocal quality, for example, listen to the difference in the sound of your voice when you have a cold.

Copyright material from Stephanie Martin (2021), *Working with Voice Disorders*, Routledge

RESONANCE

Exercises to encourage awareness of nasal release of air

A   Make a nasal sound /mm/ with your lips closed and relaxed

• Keep your throat relaxed.

• Feel a 'tingle' in your lips.

• Now make an oral sound /ah/.

• Feel the difference at the back of your nose and throat as your muscles open for the /mm/ sound and allow air into your nose.

• Make an /ah/ sound, becoming aware of the difference.

• Try to encourage the /mm/ sound to be as resonant as possible. Do not hold back.

• Make the sounds alternately /mm/ /ah/ /mm/ /ah/.

• Now try to move smoothly from /mm/ to /ah/ and say /mah/.

• Try the following nonsense words:

mah	moh	mee	may	maw	moo
ngah	ngoh	ngee	ngay	ngawn	ngoo
nah	noh	nee	nay	naw	noo

As you say these sounds, think about how the air is moving through your nose and try to make the /mm/ strong and resonant to lead you into the rest of the nonsense word.

B   Try the following single words and again remember the strong resonant /mm/ at the beginning

moon	many	money	much
mane	must	melon	mega
marsh	mole	musk	maze
mellow	mill	moan	moat

As you say these words think about how the air is moving through your nose.

Copyright material from Stephanie Martin (2021), *Working with Voice Disorders*, Routledge

RESONANCE

C **Now try the following short phrases. Try to sustain the resonant voice quality for the entire sentence**

My mum says it's OK to do my homework at nine o'clock.

Neil won't come in and he's getting very wet.

Marion is going home at ten tonight but she's coming back again tomorrow.

Many men make much money on Mondays.

My name is written on the old mailing list.

Molly seems like a nice name.

May I make macaroni, Millicent?

Mary, I went to Malta for the most of May.

Copyright material from Stephanie Martin (2021), *Working with Voice Disorders*, Routledge

BREATHING AND VOICE WORKOUT

Exercises need to be practised regularly so that the muscle control is transferred to unconscious and spontaneous control.

Quick release of tension technique

This can be done while sitting. Contrast tense and contracted muscles with tension-free muscles, enabling a more relaxed posture and alignment. Once you have released tension, try to maintain a balanced level of tension and release as you move around. Use tension-release exercises to increase your awareness of muscle tension and bring it into your control.

A   Gentle massage of the face and neck

- Carry out these exercises regularly to release tension from the muscles of the face and neck. In gentle circular movements, massage your temples above your ear and work gently down in front of your ear and along the edge of the jaw line.

- Stroke your cheeks in a downwards direction five times, firstly with your mouth closed, then allowing the jaw to gently open in a downward (not sideways) motion.

- Stretch your tongue to the right-hand side of your upper teeth (on the outside), slowly run your tongue along the outside of your teeth to the left-hand side. Repeat on your lower teeth, feeling the stretch in your jaw and tongue.

- Using your thumbs, gently massage the area under your chin.

- In a circular motion, gently massage down either side of your Adam's apple.

Copyright material from Stephanie Martin (2021), *Working with Voice Disorders*, Routledge

BREATHING AND VOICE WORKOUT

B   Exercises for posture and alignment

- Stand with your feet shoulder-width apart, keeping your knees and hip joints flexible and not locked.

- Stretch your arms up towards the ceiling and relax.

- Stretch one arm then the other towards the ceiling, then relax.

- Stretch up again and feel the stretch at your ribcage.

- Loosen your shoulders by rotating them gently.

- Move your head gently from side to side.

- 'Stand tall' – feel the spine is stretched and relax.

Copyright material from Stephanie Martin (2021), *Working with Voice Disorders*, Routledge

BREATHING AND VOICE WORKOUT

Breathing exercises

A   Diaphragmatic breathing and improved airflow control

- Sit in a tension-free position, let your breathing slow down and become shallow. Keep your shoulders and upper chest free from tension and still.

- Breathe out as fully as you can and feel your muscles contract around your lower chest and ribcage. Maintain an erect but tension-free posture.

- Slowly breathe in and feel your lungs inflate at the level of your lower chest and ribcage. Breathe out slowly on a sigh and feel the muscles and ribs return to a resting position.

- Breathe normally for several breaths.

- Repeat the above.

B   Control of outgoing airflow

- Breathe in slowly again as above.

- Breathe out and say a long /s/ sound, keeping it steady and fairly loud. Prolong it for 10+ seconds if you can. Feel your muscles control your breathing.

- Relax and breathe normally.

- Repeat this on the sound /sh/ and try to control it for 10 seconds.

- Relax and breathe normally.

C   Variations in outgoing airflow

- As above, breathe in slowly.

- Breathe out and say /s/, beginning quietly and getting louder and louder.

- Relax and breathe normally.

- Repeat this on a /sh/ sound.

- Relax and breathe normally.

- Try these two sounds with increasing loudness, decreasing loudness, then increasing to a peak of loudness and decreasing again.

- These patterns of breathing are necessary for all our spoken communication and mirror what is required for normal phrases and sentences.

Copyright material from Stephanie Martin (2021), *Working with Voice Disorders*, Routledge

BREATHING AND VOICE WORKOUT

Release of vocal tract constriction

Try all of these to see which gives the most sensation of widening and relaxation of your throat. Then focus on the one which helps most.

- *Smelling flowers/perfume/aftershave* – imagine you are smelling flowers, a lovely perfume or aftershave. You breathe in the aroma slowly and deeply through your nose. As you do this, feel your throat widen and constriction reduce.

- *Pleasant surprise* – imagine someone has arrived with a gift for you, quite unexpectedly. You express your surprise by taking in a breath, in amazement. As you take in a breath, feel your throat open and constriction reducing. Try to feel the difference from the usual tension in the vocal tract.

- *Deep sigh* – let yourself sigh loudly as if you are very tired.

- *Yawn* – let yourself yawn but keep your mouth closed to inhibit it. Feel the stretch in your throat and then relax slowly.

- *Drink* – holding an imaginary glass or large mug, tip the contents slowly over the back of the tongue and down the throat, feel the additional space that has been created.

- *Yoga Lion stretch* – the Yoga Lion: suddenly (and simultaneously) stretch fingers with eyes wide open while stretching the tongue out of the mouth. Hold the position briefly and then gently release; the jaw and tongue will slowly return to their natural positions where they remain free of tension and neutral. Experience the space inside the mouth and the back of the throat.

- *Touch of sound* – place one hand in the centre of the body over the diaphragm and breathe out silently onto an imaginary mirror held in your other hand as if you were misting up the mirror. Make sure that the breath enters and leaves the body silently.

Copyright material from Stephanie Martin (2021), *Working with Voice Disorders*, Routledge

BREATHING AND VOICE WORKOUT

Resonance balance and voice projection

- As you breathe out, maintain a sustained /m/ on a comfortable pitch. Try to start the sound like /hmm/ with a long /h/ to soften the beginning.

- As you say /hmm/ again, try to feel tingling on your lips and nose from the vibrated air inside. This indicates correct resonance balance.

- Say the word 'my' with a long and humming /m/ at the beginning.

- Do the same on these words, keeping the /m/ long and humming to bring correct resonance balance:

mine   main   moon   moan

Copyright material from Stephanie Martin (2021), *Working with Voice Disorders*, Routledge

BREATHING AND VOICE WORKOUT

Voice projection

- Ensure you are free from tension, your posture is balanced and you are breathing as described.

- Lengthen the sound 'hi' as if saying 'hiya' slowly.

- Try to say these phrases with correct breathing and with moderate volume of voice, exaggerating the intonation:

  How are you?   Who is it?   Why not?   Where did she go?

- Speak aloud or read as if you are reading to a child. Use an exaggerated intonation pattern throughout.

- Decide on a short phrase which you might use often and say it with increased volume of voice.

- Remember to apply all the techniques of good breathing and relaxed vocal tract from previous exercises.

- Try this on longer phrases and with increasing volume.

Remember that voice projection is not just about loud volume:

- Use emphasis.

- Vary your pitch.

- Articulate clearly.

- Speak more slowly.

- Face your listeners.

Copyright material from Stephanie Martin (2021), *Working with Voice Disorders*, Routledge

BREATHING AND VOICE WORKOUT

Warm-up/warm-down exercises for the voice

Try to do some of each of the exercises already included to warm up or warm down your voice. Ideally a warm up involves some exercises for:

- tension release – the whole body, the neck, shoulders, face, jaw and vocal tract;

- posture – balance and alignment;

- breathing technique and control;

- vocal tract release of tension;

- balanced resonance;

- voice production, pitch range and voice projection.

The following short warm-up exercise gives you an example of how the warm up incorporates all of the above.

Start by working on exercises to loosen up your body

- Gently push your shoulder blades together and feel the 'opening' of the front of your chest as you do so. Do this three times.

- Lift your shoulders slightly and then release them. Do this three or four times.

- Using two fingers of your right or left hand gently push your chin into your neck and feel the stretch of your muscles down the back of your neck. Do this three times.

- Imagine that your head is balanced on the top of your spine on a greasy ball bearing.

- Move the head very smoothly in a nodding 'yes' motion.

Copyright material from Stephanie Martin (2021), *Working with Voice Disorders*, Routledge

BREATHING AND VOICE WORKOUT

Move on to exercises to loosen your jaw

- Take your hands up to your cheekbones and gently stroke the jaw downwards allowing the muscles to release and lengthen.

- Imagine that the jaw is heavy and let its weight carry the jaw downwards. Monitor whether your teeth are clenched; if they are, release the tension and feel the separation of the top and bottom teeth.

Breathing out

- Sigh out to a count of five on an /ff/. When the lungs 'empty' simply allow them to refill.

- Sigh out on a count of six on a /ss/. Repeat the refill process.

- Sigh out on a count of seven on a /th/. Repeat the refill process.

- Sigh out on a count of eight on a /sh/. Repeat the refill process.

Moving the voice

- Hum any familiar tune. Purse the lips as you hum and maintain space between the upper and lower teeth in order to encourage the voice to be placed forward on the lips and in the mask of the face.

- Siren from your lowest note to your highest note using the sound /n/ or /ng/

Lips and tongue

- Purse the lips and then circle them first one way and then the other. Start at the right-hand corner of your mouth circle to the left-hand corner and then up towards your nose. Reverse the action.

- Repeat the same action with the tongue and make sure you stretch it and attempt to complete the full circle without missing out any section.

As you go through the different stages of the warm up do make sure you continue to monitor any tension that may creep in at any point.

Copyright material from Stephanie Martin (2021), *Working with Voice Disorders*, Routledge

GLOBUS AND CHRONIC COUGH

Globus

As mentioned in Chapter 2, it is imperative that the feeling of a lump in the throat is fully investigated to ensure that there is no physical cause requiring further assessment or intervention. Laryngopharyngeal or gastro-pharyngeal reflux must be considered as a potential cause and treatment instigated if necessary. Once a physical cause has been excluded or treated, the following therapy suggestions can be tried.

- Voice care advice is imperative to reduce, and ultimately eradicate, throat clearing; ensure adequate hydration and avoidance of irritants. See Appendix I: Voice Care Advice.

- Use exercises to reduce vocal tract constriction.

- Select voice production exercises to alleviate any excess effort in the laryngeal musculature.

- Patients should aim to replace throat clearing and symptoms of tension with release of constriction and good voice production techniques.

Chronic cough

Irritation in the vocal tract is frequently an early symptom of a muscle tension dysphonia. Therefore, the advice relating to irritation is relevant to chronic cough once physical causes, which can be treated, have been eliminated or medication prescribed:

- voice care advice,

- breathing techniques,

- release of constriction.

The aim should be to anticipate the cough response and replace this with release of constriction and controlled breathing.

- Voice production exercises to alleviate any excess effort in the laryngeal musculature which may exacerbate irritation.

Copyright material from Stephanie Martin (2021), *Working with Voice Disorders*, Routledge

VOCAL CORD DYSFUNCTION

Vocal cord dysfunction

Because there is a close relationship between chronic cough and VCD, there are similarities in the suggested intervention:

- reassurance,

- relaxation and stress reduction strategies,

- voice care advice,

- breathing techniques,

- release of constriction,

- reduction of vocal tract tension through voice exercises – gentle voicing.

Copyright material from Stephanie Martin (2021), *Working with Voice Disorders*, Routledge

OUTLINE FOR VOICE INFORMATION GROUP

Programme outline

- Welcome and introduction

- Collect Voice Impact Profile questionnaires for profiles

- Housekeeping

- Purpose of the group

The normal voice

- How voice works

- The vocal folds

- Breathing

- Pitch and voice quality

- Emotion and its influence on voice

- Online resources of normal voice production

Factors affecting voice: cause, effect and how to self-help

- Tension

- Inefficient breathing

- Inadequate hydration

- Acid reflux

- Throat clearing/coughing

- Volume of voice/vocal demand

- Environmental factors

Copyright material from Stephanie Martin (2021), *Working with Voice Disorders*, Routledge

OUTLINE FOR VOICE INFORMATION GROUP

Online resources of disordered voice and vocal fold appearance and movement

Voice care and advice

Options/choices for patients

- Opt for advice only and discharge.

- Opt for advice and return for review in specified time.

- Opt for therapy programme.

- Brief personal discussion, if requested, to assist patient's decision on opt in/out.

- Check the patient's contact details and preferred time and place of therapy.

- Advise that patients may make contact in future for review, even if the opt-out option has been chosen. Open access process in place.

- Assure patients of clinician contact within a specified period to arrange further appointments.

Copyright material from Stephanie Martin (2021), *Working with Voice Disorders*, Routledge

OUTLINE FOR A THREE-HOUR TEACHERS' WORKSHOP

Programme outline

- Welcome and introduction

- Housekeeping

- Purpose of the group

The normal voice

- How voice works

- The vocal folds

- Breathing

- Pitch and voice quality

- Emotion and its influence on voice

- Online resources of normal voice production

Factors affecting the teaching voice: cause, effect and how to self-help

- Posture and tension

- Inefficient breathing

- Inadequate hydration

- Acid reflux

- Throat clearing/coughing

- Volume of voice/vocal demand

- Environmental factors

Copyright material from Stephanie Martin (2021), *Working with Voice Disorders*, Routledge

OUTLINE FOR A THREE-SESSION TEACHERS' WORKSHOP

Online resources of disordered voice and vocal fold appearance and movement

Voice care and advice

Practical exercise session of 1–1.5 hours

- Release of tension

- Posture

- Breathing

- Release of constriction

- Gentle voicing

- Voice projection

Copyright material from Stephanie Martin (2021), *Working with Voice Disorders*, Routledge

OUTLINE FOR A THREE-SESSION TEACHERS' WORKSHOP

Programme outline - session 1: You and your voice

Discussion

- Facts and figures regarding voice problems

- Negative impact factors - 'the worst things you can do for your voice'

- Early warning signs

- Voice care and advice

- Diaphragmatic breathing

Practical session

- Release of tension

- Posture

- Airflow control

Tasks

- Goal - change two things about your voice use

- Write in two goals/targets from the pack

- Practise five minutes every day on release of tension and breathing

- Try to increase your sentence length on one breath.

Copyright material from Stephanie Martin (2021), *Working with Voice Disorders*, Routledge

OUTLINE FOR A THREE-SESSION TEACHERS' WORKSHOP

Programme outline – session 2: Workplace challenges for your voice

Discussion

- Feedback from tasks

- Vocal loading and recovery time

- Stress and self-management for voice

- Posture and alignment

- Acoustics and dead spots

Practical session

- Release of tension – imagery

- Deconstriction

- Review of breathing exercises and posture

- Voice projection

Tasks

- Voice diary – write up for one week or longer

- Analyse the acoustics of your classroom and adapt them if possible/necessary

- Choose one postural problem – try to consistently improve/alter this

- Review all exercises regularly

- Prompt – bring a question for next session's question box

Copyright material from Stephanie Martin (2021), *Working with Voice Disorders*, Routledge

OUTLINE FOR A THREE-SESSION TEACHERS' WORKSHOP

Programme outline – session 3: Bringing it all together

Discussion

- Feedback from previous tasks

- General feedback on programme and impact

- Problem solving – What's wrong with their voice? What are they doing wrong?

- Negative practice – tension, rate and clarity

- Projection – have fun with your voice

- How loud can you be? What is 'twang'?

Question time

- Fill up the question box

Tasks

- Decide on a prompt to help you remember your voice techniques

- Read the pack thoroughly

- Practise all your exercises regularly

- Try to apply the techniques of voice in everyday situations

The outlines above for the breathing and voice workout, the voice information group and the teachers' workshops have been used extensively by the author and colleagues. While they are comprehensive, they are clearly not the only approach to group planning. However, it is hoped that the outlines will provide a starting point for discussion and planning in a format that suits the needs of the groups and the available resources.

Copyright material from Stephanie Martin (2021), *Working with Voice Disorders*, Routledge

8

SHAPING THE FUTURE

Introduction

As with all dynamic areas of medicine, change is continuous and Speech and Language Therapy is not immune to change. Many aspects of service provision and clinical skills are subject to rapid change and evolution, which impacts on the work of the clinician involved in delivering a service to patients with a voice disorder. The following pages consider a number of professional issues that may well affect the work of clinicians in the field of voice disorders in the coming years.

Service provision

One concept that has already been challenged and may indeed need to be further challenged in terms of voice therapy is the concept of voice work being undertaken on an individual rather than on a group basis (Almeida *et al.*, 2015).

Previous chapters have outlined the Voice Information Group (VIG) as a means of first contact with patients. This allows a number of patients with voice disorders to be seen together, giving each patient an opportunity to decide which option for further intervention – advice or therapy – best suits their lifestyle. Clinical audit of the use of VIGs demonstrates the clinical efficiency of this approach in optimal use of staffing, time and financial resources (Lockhart, 2011; Burt and Fletcher, 2019).

A clinical efficiencies audit of one VIG specialist voice service in Lanarkshire, Scotland was conducted over a 12-month period (2009–2010). A total of 351 patients were appointed to VIGs during this time, with between five and ten patients in each group. Patients known to have a vocal fold paresis or paralysis, neurological conditions, those with pre-cancerous lesions or a diagnosis of cancer were not included but were given individual appointments. Using this VIG model, between 180 and 200 treatment slots were released, which would have been allocated for individual patient assessment or treatment, equalling over 60 treatment sessions.

By employing the VIG as the first contact in a group format, resources of clinical time were released and wastage of clinical sessions due to patients' failure to attend were minimised. Of those who attended, 40% of patients opted for voice therapy, 12% for advice and review and 8% opted to apply advice and be discharged. The remaining 40% did not attend the first appointment offered, but took up different options: opted to reappoint to a more suitable time, requested an individual appointment for various reasons, decided to cancel their appointment as unnecessary or failed to attend. Almost 100% of patients who attended VIGs rated their experience positively in an evaluation questionnaire, compliance in attendance was almost 100% for return visits, and patients were well motivated to self-management.

For those attending for therapy or opting to apply advice and attend for a review appointment, patient experience evaluations showed an average of 92% satisfaction with the service, the group format and the options provided. Moreover, return visits after applying advice for three to four months resulted in 'on average' two to five sessions required for further intervention. Thereafter, the patient was discharged from the service as having attained a satisfactory result in terms of acceptable and functional voice quality and a good outcome from laryngeal examination.

It is therefore the view of the author that where there is a need for clinical efficiency savings and best use of resources, the VIG model is highly appropriate for voice-disordered patients and is valuable in demonstrating clinical efficiency, best use of clinical capacity and skill mix (Simberg *et al.*, 2006). Studies suggest group therapy is a positive experience as it operates with health promotion aspects from the construction of concepts and notions of self-care and health education, and offers therapeutic intervention possibilities in which the individual is assisted with a biopsychosocial approach (Almeida *et al.*, 2015). It is also important to consider the value that group attendance has in increasing motivation, changing behaviour and achieving improvement through the experience of being part of a group who shared similar experiences and challenges (Maclean *et al.*, 2000; Sandlund, 2018).

Endoscopic evaluation of the larynx (EEL)

The recent development of a clear and comprehensive framework for clinicians with reference to EEL has been published by the Royal College of Speech and Language Therapists and is to be welcomed. Entitled 'RCSLT competency framework and training log. Speech and Language Therapy endoscopic evaluation of the larynx (EEL) for clinical voice disorders, competency framework and training log' and developed by specialist and highly specialist clinicians, it is available on line (www.rcslt.org) and includes extensive commentary and guidelines for clinicians. It is beyond the remit of this book to include extensive comment on EEL, but the author highly recommends that in addition to this resource, readers go to 'Laryngeal Endoscopy and Voice Therapy' (2016) by the lead author of the RCSLT framework, Sue Jones, for guidance and direction.

The document states:

> EEL is an established procedure in both ENT and speech and language therapy practice for
> the assessment and differential diagnosis of voice disorders. More recently, EEL has become

a standard tool for assessing laryngopharyngeal gesture and trialing therapy techniques in voice disorders, as well as providing biofeedback during therapy sessions. As ENT/speech and language therapy practice has evolved, and as SLTs have taken on the role of advanced/expert clinical practitioners in clinical voice disorders, the use of EEL by SLTs has been extended in both the types of voice clinics undertaken independently and in the use of EEL as a therapeutic tool.

Within the document the authors address a number of issues, such as why a competency framework is needed. It is needed, they suggest, in order to address the skills and competencies that are required by SLTs performing EEL. It is a UK-wide document aimed to cover all situations in which an SLT may perform EEL, including working within a joint clinic directly with ear, nose and throat (ENT) teams and in more independent capacities working autonomously but still within an agreed framework with ENT consultants. The expectation is that SLTs working through this competency framework will already be practising confidently and competently with clinical voice disorders at a specialist level. The framework will bring together knowledge and practical competencies and will be in use throughout the SLT's career. Signed evidence of skill acquisition and maintenance will be provided, either through independent activity or through the verification of an appropriately skilled supervisor. The document is seen as a training and competency framework for SLTs who perform EEL for the purpose of assessing and managing clinical voice disorders and will be a useful resource to record ongoing learning and development, which would fit within the annual appraisal process of most organisations. Not only will it provide guidance as to training and levels of competencies needed to work at specific levels as an endoscopy practitioner, it will also provide guidance to the Health and Care Professions Council (HCPC), managers, postgraduate training providers, students, clinicians and clinical leaders. The document will help to guide services, ensuring that EEL is performed by practitioners with the appropriate skills in a safe clinical environment.

This framework was temporarily superseded by a RCSLT guidance document ('Aerosol generating procedures, dysphagia assessment and COVID-19: a rapid review', first published 1 June 2020; https://doi.org/10.1111/1460-6984.12544). This takes account of changes required in SLT-led endoscopic procedures during the COVID-19 pandemic. A return to the guidance document will obviously depend on the outcome of the pandemic. The RCSLT COVID-19 Advisory Group has guidance for clinicians while the pandemic lasts, and while it is difficult to speculate how working practices will alter post pandemic, it would not be unreasonable to think that there may indeed be a need to make further changes to the framework depending on the situation at that time.

Post COVID-19

The world pandemic brought rapid change to clinical working, changes which are likely to impact on the work of the clinician in delivering a service to patients within respiratory medicine and ENT voice therapy. As a result of the COVID-19 virus clinicians will be dealing with a number of patients with specific voice problems as a result of the virus and comorbid issues resulting from intubation. The RCSLT issued guidance regarding issues of personal care and protection equipment for clinicians working with patients and the reader is advised to look online for up-to-date information. The British Laryngological Association has an advice sheet offering advice for patients who experienced voice problems after COVID-19 prepared by a team of UK Specialist Speech and Language Therapists which is very useful. As more is known about the virus and there is more robust research available, clinicians will be much better informed and preparation for another pandemic/epidemic will find that resources are more readily available. In the short term, advice for vocal hygiene and recognition of the known links between emotion and the voice and what patients may require in terms of emotional recovery and support is the most efficacious intervention and these should be followed. In recognition of the emotional toll the pandemic has exerted on both patients and staff, Public Health England has produced a COVID-19 Psychological First Aid free online course under the auspices of FutureLearn. It is to be recommended for those dealing with the public during the pandemic, although it is not time-sensitive and provides very useful and helpful advice and is to be recommended for those who are working with those in psychological distress. As COVID-19 patients recover from extended periods in critical care with many days of intubation, the work of a decade ago (Nixon *et al.*, 2010) comes into sharp focus. In their study, 33% of patients admitted to intensive care reported a degree of vocal morbidity greater than that suffered by patients treated for early laryngeal cancer. Sixteen per cent of patients reported a degree of morbidity greater than that suffered by patients attending voice clinics and up to one-third of patients who survived admission to an intensive care unit reported suffering significant vocal morbidity. The most common complication of prolonged endotracheal intubation is vocal change with an instance of hoarseness varying widely from 14% to 50% (Kiran *et al.*, 2016). While the hoarseness is mostly temporary, incidents of arytenoid dislocation varies between 1 in 1000 and 1 in 4000 in various studies (Yamanaka *et al.*, 2009), with an increased risk of arytenoid dislocation occurring in patients with laryngomalacia and in those on chronic steroid therapy (Rubin *et al.*, 2005). Given the number of patients intubated for long periods with COVID-19, it is likely that the number of voice patients presenting with post-intubation hoarseness will have increased exponentially. There is also early evidence that the pulmonary damage incurred as a result of COVID-19 may leave patients with long-lasting irreversible pulmonary insult, such as pulmonary fibrosis, the legacy of which may lead to increasing numbers of patients presenting in ENT clinics.

Telehealth

Telemedicine is not new, it is a term coined in the 1970s, which literally means 'healing at a distance'. Telemedicine is an open and constantly evolving science, as it incorporates new technological advances and responds and adapts to the changing health needs and contexts of societies. Telemedicine will profoundly transform the delivery of health services in the industrialised world by migrating healthcare delivery away from hospitals and clinics into homes.

The term telemedicine was at one time restricted to services delivered by doctors, while telehealth signified services provided by health professionals in general, but that distinction has now largely been discontinued and the terms telemedicine and telehealth are often used interchangeably, but telehealth has evolved to encapsulate a broader array of digital healthcare activities and services.

The World Health Organisation (WHO) adopted the following broad description of Telehealth as:

> the delivery of health care services, where patients and providers are separated by distance. Telehealth uses ICT for the exchange of information for the diagnosis and treatment of diseases and injuries, research and evaluation, and for the continuing education of health professionals. Telehealth can contribute to achieving universal health coverage by improving access for patients to quality, cost-effective, health services wherever they may be. It is particularly valuable for those in remote areas, vulnerable groups and ageing populations. (WHO, 1998)

Telehealth has four main purposes, namely:

- to provide clinical support,
- to connect users who are not in the same physical location,
- to use various types of information and communication technology (ICT) in therapy to connect clinician and patient,
- to improve health outcomes.

The biggest drivers of telemedicine over the past decade have been the increasing availability and utilisation of ICTs by the general population, rapidly creating new possibilities for healthcare service and delivery on a world-wide basis. The Internet has expanded the scope of telemedicine to encompass web-based applications and multimedia approaches online and has enabled healthcare providers to implement new and more efficient ways of providing care.

The potential impact of telehealth on voice therapy is considerable as it allows information to be transmitted on either a store and forward (asynchronous) or real-time (synchronous) basis. In both synchronous and asynchronous telemedicine, relevant information may be transmitted in a variety of media, such as text, audio, video, or still images.

The challenge for clinicians is to determine which diagnostic and therapeutic procedures are adaptable to distance interaction and which are not, and to identify which clinical populations are appropriate to evaluate and treat remotely and which are not. For example, manual circumlaryngeal techniques would not be an option in treating muscle tension dysphonia remotely because it requires the clinician to palpate and manipulate the patient's larynx. On the other hand, vocal rehabilitation counselling to eliminate phonotraumatic behaviours has good potential to be accomplished successfully remotely. Fu *et al.* (2015) delivered intensive voice therapy via videoconferencing to ten women with vocal nodules and found significant improvement in perceptual, vocal fold function, acoustic and physiological parameters as well as nodule sizes and life post-treatment. All participants were highly positive about their experience. In the delivery of intensive voice therapy for vocal fold nodules via telepractice, Rangarathnam *et al.* (2015) investigated the utility of telepractice for delivering flow phonation exercises to two groups of patients with primary muscle tension dysphonia (MTD). Results for the two service delivery groups, telepractice and standard therapy, were comparable, with no significant differences observed for perceptual and quality-of-life measures. The researchers concluded that the provision of behavioural treatment to patients with MTD was successful. An online telepractice model for the prevention of voice disorders in vocally healthy student teachers demonstrated success in preventative voice work with student teachers, evaluated by a smartphone application (Grillo *et al.*, 2017).

Another aspect to consider is whether a telehealth model may be more appropriate at different phases of therapy. If therapy techniques need to be established in the traditional model of clinical intervention, perhaps generalisation and maintenance of voice could be facilitated and monitored remotely. Mashima *et al.* (2003) compared the telehealth model with the conventional model of delivering voice therapy and found no significant differences between remotely and conventionally delivered voice therapy for the following outcomes: perception of voice quality, acoustic changes, patient satisfaction, and laryngeal changes. Two studies looking at treating patients with Parkinson's disease had positive outcomes. Howell *et al.* (2009) undertook a feasibility study delivering the Lee Silverman Voice Treatment (LSVT) by web camera and Constantinescu *et al.* (2011) treated disordered speech and voice in Parkinson's disease online.

The embargo on travel and social distancing imposed during the 2019/20 pandemic has thrown telemedicine into sharper focus. As the recent pandemic underlined, telehealth has considerable value to voice patients who cannot travel due to travel restrictions, or indeed in more 'normal' times it has application for those patients who may not have a centre of excellence nearby or may lack the services of a specialist clinician, as is the case for transgender patients who cannot, for example, access Gender Identity Clinics in their area and need to travel to a centre of excellence at considerable financial, physical and emotional cost. Major financial savings have been realised by the use of telehealth (Towey, 2012; Radford and Davies, 2020). Even though low-cost telemedicine applications have proven to be feasible, clinically useful, sustainable and scalable, these applications do not, in the case of working with voice-disordered patients, appear to have previously been adopted on a significant scale. As with all patient-clinician interaction, issues pertaining to confidentiality, dignity and privacy are of ethical concern with respect to telemedicine. It is imperative that treatment is implemented equitably and to the highest ethical standards, to ensure no marginalisation of care. When deciding whether telehealth is appropriate to use and where local guidelines do not exist, appropriateness for telehealth should be determined on a case-by-case basis with selections firmly based on:

- the client's cognitive, physical, or perceptual impairments;
- consideration as to what family, carer or teaching support the client has available to them to support their access to the technology;
- clinical judgement;
- the client's informed choice;
- professional standards of care.

Services via telehealth will need to be carefully considered and it may be that modifications need to be made to the treatment material, therapy techniques, equipment and the setting. The RCSLT has Telehealth Guidance on their website and readers are recommended to look there for further information. In 2019, the special interest group on ASHA published a report on building a successful Voice Telepractice Programme which is also of interest. In the UK the National Health Service (NHS) has online resources such as implementation toolkits which offer advice and resources to explore the use of online consultations in primary care. While these may not directly resonate with clinicians working with voice disorders, it is a valuable source of information if approaching telehealth for the first time. The National Institute for Health Research conducted a very interesting research project called VOCAL: Virtual Online Consultations– Advantages and Limitations, www.vocalproject.co.uk (Greenhalgh *etal.*, 2016) which looked at video outpatient consultations (via Skype) based in two clinical settings in an NHS acute trust in London. The researchers looked at the clinician and patient inter-action during consultations through the use of audio, video and screen capture to produce rich multimodal data on 30 virtual consultations. They mapped the administrative and clin-ical processes that needed to change to implement and support the Skype consultations. In addition, they conducted interviews with national stakeholders in order to understand the national-level context for the introduction of virtual consultations in NHS organisations and what measures might incentivise and make them easier. Their findings indicated that when clinical, technical and practical preconditions were met, video consultations appeared safe and were popular with some patients and staff; the consultations were very slightly shorter and patients did slightly more talking than compared with face-to-face talking, and the consultations worked better when the clinician and patient already knew and trusted each other. The evidence base on remote consultations by video technology is accumu-lating and the complex challenges of delivering healthcare to an ageing and increasingly diverse population suggest that alternatives to current consultation models are needed. Studies in education and in speech and language therapy have promoted the view that remote consultation, if carefully assessed and managed with sufficient safe-guarding and risk assessment undertaken, should provide, under certain conditions, a confident alterna-tive for the clinician when working with voice disorders.

Summary

To end, as the book began, with the truism that voice is a critical indicator of both physio-logical and psychological well-being and as such offers a particularly acute and effective gauge of physical and mental health. For that reason, the clinician's assessment and appraisal of the patient should include an assessment of a constellation of factors in the patient's life – emotional, anatomical, physiological, genetic, cognitive, environmental and mechanical – all of which may have contributed to the predisposing, precipitating, perpetu-ating and present factors in the patient's voice disorder.

One aspect, however, which often fails to be considered is the contribution that the clinician's own vocal production may make to treatment outcomes. Aspects of adherence and compliance have already been considered in a previous chapter, but the vocal quality and voice use that the clinician models is rarely considered. This is in no way to suggest that those working in the field of voice require a level of voice use that would comply with that of an Elite Voice User (Koufman, 1998). Nevertheless, in the author's opinion it is important to have achieved a degree of vocal ability that will provide patients with a model that elicits confidence in the clinician's own vocal repertoire and allows the patient to recognize that the clinician fully understands and appreciates how vocal change can be achieved. The clinician is therefore demonstrating skills to model a range of vocal settings, from imbalanced resonance to supralaryngeal constriction, and can therefore appreciate what and where problems may exist and can offer practical exemplars from which to work. Indeed, when working with professional voice users, providing a good vocal model is an acknowledgement that the clinician understands their occupational vocal demands. It is the author's view, therefore, that clinicians working with voice disorders should be able to model all of the exercises contained within this book and would encourage clinicians to this end.

Throughout this book, the author's goal has been to provide a comprehensive and practical approach to voice disorders. The content reflects a strong clinical bias and confidence in the tried-and-tested materials provided. The author is privileged to work in a field that is fulfilling, stimulating, interesting and endlessly rewarding, and the hope is that all those who read this book will be encouraged to pursue the challenges inherent in working with voice disorders.

As Denis Podalydes says, 'The voice makes you aware of people because spirit, intellect, psyche are integrated and embodied in the voice' (Abberton, 2009).

Bibliography

Abberton E (2009) 'Don't look at me in that tone of voice!' Gunnar Rugheimer lecture of the BVA.

Abitbol J (2006) *Odyssey of the Voice*, Plural Publishing, San Diego, CA.

Age UK (2015) 'Evidence review loneliness in later life'. www.ageuk.org.uk/globalassets/age-uk/ documents/reports-and-publications/reports-and-briefings/health-wellbeing/rb_june15_ lonelines_in_later_life_evidence_review.pdf.

Ahmed N, Ellins J, Krelle H & Lawrie M. (2014) *Person Centred Care: From Ideas to Action*, Health Foundation, London.

Allen J, Nouraur RSA & Sandhu GS (2019) *A Case Based Approach*, Plural Publishing, San Diego, CA.

Almeida L, Fahning A, Trajano F, Anjos U *et al.* (2015) 'Group voice therapy and its effectiveness in the treatment of dysphonia: a systematic review'. *CEFAC*, 17, pp. 2000-8.

Altman KW (2007) 'Vocal fold masses'. *Otolaryngologic Clinics of North America*, 40, 1091-108.

Ambizas EM & Etzel JV (2017) 'Proton Pump Inhibitors: Considerations with long terms use'. *US Pharmacist*, 42(7), pp. 4-7.

American Geriatrics Society Expert Panel on PCC (2015) 'Person centred care: A definition and essential elements'. *Journal of the American Geriatrics Society*, December 2.

Amir O & Biron-Shental T (2004) 'The impact of hormonal fluctuations on female vocal folds'. *Current Opinion in Otolaryngology & Head and Neck Surgery*, 12, pp. 180-4.

Amir O, Biron-Shental T, Muchnik C & Kishon-Rabin L (2003) 'Do oral contraceptives improve voice quality? Limited trial on low-dose formulations'. *Obstetrics & Gynecology*, 101, pp. 773-7.

Andrews ML (2006) *Manual of Voice Treatment*, Singular Publishing Group, San Diego, CA.

Andrus JG & Shapshay SM (2006) 'Contemporary management of laryngeal papilloma in adults and children'. *Otolaryngologic Clinics of North America*, 39, pp. 135-58.

Appleby BS & Rosenburg PB (2006) 'Aerophagia as the initial presenting symptom of a depressed patient'. *Journal of Clinical Psychiatry*, 8 (4), pp245-6.

Aronson AE (1985) *Clinical Voice Disorders; an interdisciplinary approach*, 3rd edn, Thieme, New York.

Aronson AE (1990a) *Clinical Voice Disorders; an interdisciplinary approach*, 4th edn, Thieme, New York.

Aronson AE (1990b) 'Importance of the psychosocial interview in the diagnosis and treatment of "functional" voice disorders'. *Journal of Voice*, 4, pp. 287-89.

Assmann (2013) 'Efficacy Study of Botulinum Toxin (BOTOX) injections to Treat Vocal Fold Granulomas'. Clinical Trials.gov Identifier: NCTO16678053 2012-2017.

Baker J (2010) 'Women's voices: lost or mislaid, stolen or strayed?' *International Journal of Speech-Language Pathology*, 12(2), pp. 94-106.

Baker, J. (2017) *Psychological Perspectives on the Management of Voice Disorders*, Compton Publishers, Oxford.

Baker J, Ben-Tovim DI, Butcher A, Esterman A & McLaughlin K (2007) 'Development of a modified diagnostic classification system for voice disorders with interrater reliability study'. *Logopedics Phoniatrics Vocology*, 32(3), pp. 99-112.

Bassiouny S (1998) 'Efficacy of the accent method of voice therapy'. *Folia Phonatrica et Logopedica*, 50, pp. 146-64.

Behlau M, Oliveira G & Pontes P (2009) 'Vocal fold self-disruption after phonotrauma on a lead actor: a case presentation'. *Journal of Voice*, 23(6), pp. 726-32.

Behrman A & Sulica L (2003) 'Voice rest after microlaryngoscopy: current opinion and practice', *Laryngoscope*, 113(12), pp. 2182-6.

Belafsky PC, Postma GN, Reylbach TR, Holland BW & Koufman JA (2002) 'Muscle tension dysphonia as a sign of underlying glottal insufficiency'. *Otolaryngology – Head & Neck Surgery*, 127(5), pp. 448-5i.

Bhalla RK, Watson G, Taylor W, Jones AS & Roland NJ (2009) 'Acoustic analysis in asthmatics and the influence of inhaled corticosteroid therapy'. *Journal of Voice*, 23(4), pp. 505-11.

Bibby JRL, Cotton SM, Perry A & Corry JF (2007) 'Voice outcomes after radiotherapy treatment for early glottic cancer: assessment using multidimensional tools'. *Head & Neck*, 30, pp. 600-10.

Birring SS, Prudon B, Carr AJ, Singh SJ, Morgan MDL & Pavord ID (2003) 'Development of a symptom specific health status measure for patients with chronic cough: Leicester Cough Questionnaire (LCQ)'. *Thorax*, 58, pp. 339-43.

Bless D & Hirano M (1982) 'Verbal instructions: a critical variable in obtaining optimal performance for maximum phonation time'. Paper presented at ASHA Convention, Toronto, Canada.

Boehme G & Gross M (2005) *Stroboscopy*, Whurr, London.

Boersma P & Weenink DJM (2001) 'Praat, a system for doing phonetics by computer'. *Glot International*, 5(9/10), pp. 341-5.

Boone DR & McFarlane SC (1988) *The Voice and Voice Therapy*, 4th edn, Prentice-Hall, Englewood Cliffs, NJ.

Bostrom RN (2006) 'The process of listening' in Hargie, O. (ed.), *The Handbook of Communication Skills*, 3rd edn, Routledge, London.

British Medical Journal (2012) 'Use of proton pump inhibitors and risk of hip fracture in relation to dietary and lifestyle factors: a prospective cohort study'. *British Medical Journal*, 344, e372.

British Medical Journal (2019) 'NHS prescribed record number of antidepressants last year'. *British Medical Journal*, 364, l1508.

British Voice Association (2012) 'Report on the BVA World Voice Day Questionnaire for Voice Clinics'. BVA, London, November.

Brown KK, Wingfield ER & Kimball MD (2006) 'Determining the relative importance of patient motivations for nonadherence to topical corticosteroid therapy in psoriasis'. *Journal of the American Academy of Dermatology*, 55(4), pp. 607-13.

Bruzzi C, Salsi D, Minghetti D *et al.* (2017) 'Presbyphonia'. *Acta Biomedica*, 88(1), pp. 6-10.

Buddiga P (2011) 'Vocal cord dysfunction clinical presentation'. emedicine.medscape.com/article/137782-overview

Buhl R (2006) 'Local oropharyngeal side effects of inhaled corticosteroids in patients with asthma'. *Allergy*, 61, pp. 518-26.

Bunch Dayme M (2005) *The Performer's Voice*, WW Norton & Company, New York.

Burns K (2016) *Focus on Solutions: a Health Professional's Guide*, 2nd edn, Solutions Books, London.

Burns K & Northcott S (2021) *Working with Solution Focused Brief Therapy in Health Care Settings* (in press).

Burt J & Fletcher J (2019) 'A voice for the group'. *Bulletin of the RCSLT*, 811, pp. 16-17.

Butcher P, Elias A & Cavalli L (2007) *Understanding and Treating Psychogenic Voice Disorder – a CBT framework*, John Wiley & Sons, Chichester.

Butler C (2019) 'Reflective practice risks competent clinical practice'. www.ncl.ac.uk.

Butler JE, Hammond TH & Gray SD (2001) 'Gender-related differences of hyaluronic acid distribution in the human vocal'. *The Laryngoscope*, 111(5), pp. 907-11.

Carding PN (2003) 'Voice pathology clinics in the UK'. *Clinical Otolaryngology and Allied Sciences*, 28, pp. 477-8.

Carding PN, Wilson J, MacKenzie K & Deary V (2009) 'Measuring voice outcomes: state of the science review'. *Journal of Laryngology and Otology* 123, pp. 823-9.

Carding PN, Bos-Clark M, Fu S, Gillivan Murphy P, Jones SM & Walton C (2017) 'Evaluating the efficacy of voice therapy for functional organic and neurological voice disorders'. *Clinical Otolaryngology*, 42, pp. 201–17.

Carding QVP, Carding PN, Horsley IA & Docherty GJ (1999) 'A study of the effectiveness of voice therapy in the treatment of 45 patients with nonorganic dysphonia'. *Journal of Voice*, 13(1), pp. 72–104.

Caruso S, Rocasalva L, Sapienza G, Zappala M, Nuciforo G & Biondi S (2000) 'Laryngological aspects in women with surgically induced menopause who were treated with transdermal estrogen replacement therapy'. *Fertility and Sterility*, 74, pp. 1073–9.

Catley D, Harris KJ, Mayo MS *et al.* (2006), 'Adherence to principles of motivational interviewing and client within-session behaviour'. *Behavioural and Cognitive Psychotherapy*, 34, pp. 43–56.

Cavalli L (2016) 'Voice therapy for psychogenic dysphonia evidence and practice'. Cutting Edge Conference, New Zealand.

Centers for Disease Control and Prevention (2020) 'Outbreak of lung injury associated with e-cigarette use or vaping'. www.cdc.gov/tobacco/basic_information/e-cigarettes/severe-lung-disease.html.

Chan RW, Gray SD & Titze IR (2001) 'The importance of hyaluronic acid in vocal fold biomechanics'. *Otolaryngology and Neck Surgery*, 124(6), pp. 607–14.

Chan Y, Irish JC, Wood SJ *et al.* (2002) 'Patient education and informed consent in head and neck surgery'. *Archives of Otolaryngology – Head & Neck Surgery*, 128, pp. 1269–74.

Chapman JL (2017) *Singing and Teaching of Singing*, Plural Publishing, San Diego, CA.

Chhetri DK & Mendelsohn AH (2010) 'Hyaluronic acid for the treatment of vocal fold scars'. *Current Opinion in Otolaryngology Head and Neck Surgery*, 18(6), pp. 498–502.

Chitkara DK, Bredenoord J, Rucker MJ &Talley NJ (2005) 'Aerophagia in adults: a comparison with functional dyspepsia'. *Alimentary Pharmacology & Therapeutics*, 22(9), pp. 855–8.

Cielo CA, Padilha de Moraes Lima J, Christmann MK *et al.* (2013) 'Semioccluded vocal tract exercises: literature review'. *Rev. CEFAC*, 15(6), pp. 1679–89.

Cigrang JA (2006) 'Behavioural treatment of chronic belching due to aerophagia in a normal adult'. *Behaviour Modification*, 30(3), pp. 341–51.

Collins SA (2000) 'Male voices and women's choices'. *Animal Behaviour*, 60, pp. 773–80.

Colton RH, Casper JK & Leonard RJ (2011) *Understanding Voice Problems*, 4th edn, Lippincott Williams & Wilkins, Philadelphia, PA.

Constantinescu G, Theodoros D, Russell T, Ward E, Wilson S & Wootton R (2011) 'Treating disordered speech and voice in Parkinson's disease online: a randomized controlled non-inferiority trial'. *International Journal of Language and Communication Disorders*, 46(1), pp. 1–16.

Cooper M (1973) *Modern Techniques of Vocal Rehabilitation*, Charles C. Thomas, Springfield, IL.

Cooper M & Nahum AM (1967) 'Vocal rehabilitation for contact ulcer of the larynx'. *Archives of Otolaryngology – Head & Neck Surgery*, 85(1), pp. 41–6.

Dacakis G (2000) 'Long-term maintenance of fundamental frequency increases in male-to-female transsexuals'. *Journal of Voice*, 14, pp. 549–56.

Dacakis G (2006) 'Assessment and goals', in Adler RK, Hirsh S & Mordaunt M (eds), *Voice and Communication Therapy for the Transgender/Transsexual Client*, Plural Publishing, San Diego, CA.

Dacakis, M Davies S, Oates JM *et al.* (2013) 'Development and preliminary evaluation of the Transsexual Voice Questionnaire for Male-to-Female Transsexuals'. *Journal of Voice*, 27(3), pp. 312–20.

Dagli M, Sati I, Acar A, Stone RE, Dursun G & Eryilmaz A (2008) 'Mutational falsetto: intervention outcomes in 45 patients'. *The Journal of Laryngology & Otology*, 122, pp. 277–81.

Davies S, Papp VG & Antoni C (2015) 'Voice and communication change for gender nonconforming individuals giving voice to the person inside'. *International Journal of Transgenderism*, 16, pp. 117–59.

De Jong FICRS, Kooijman PGC, Thomas G, Huinck WJ, Graamans K & Schutte HK (2006) 'Epidemiology of voice problems in Dutch teachers'. *Folia Phoniatrica et Logopaedica*, 58, pp. 186–98.

Deary IJ, Wilson JA, Carding PN & MacKenzie K (2003) 'VoiSS: a patient-derived voice symptom scale'. *Journal of Psychosomatic Research*, 54(5), pp. 483-9.

Deary V, McColl E, Carding P *et al.* (2018) 'A psychosocial intervention for the management of functional dysphonia: Complex Intervention Development and Pilot Randomised Trial'. *Pilot and Feasibility Studies*, 4, p. 46.

Deem F & Miller L (2000) *Manual of Voice Therapy*, 2nd edn, PRO-ED, Austin, TX.

Dejardins M, Halstead L, Cooke M *et al.* (2016) 'A systematic review of voice therapy: what "effectiveness" really implies'. *Journal of Voice*, 31(3), pp. 392.e13-392.e32.

Dejonckere PH, Clements P, Bradley P & Cornut G (2001) 'A basic protocol for functional assessment of voice pathology especially for investigating the efficacy of phonosurgical treatments and evaluating new assessment techniques – guideline elaborated by the Committee on Phonatrics of the European Laryngological Society'. *Archiv für Klinische und Experimentelle Ohren-Nasen-und Kehikopfheilkunde*, 258(2), pp. 77-82.

Denizoglu I & Sihvo M (2010) 'LaxVox voice therapy technique'. *Current Practise in Otolaryngology, Rhinology & Laryngology*, 6(2), pp. 284-95yh.

Devaney KO, Rinaldo A & Ferlito A (2005) 'Vocal process granuloma of the larynx – recognition, differential diagnosis and treatment'. *Oral Oncology*, 41, pp. 666-9.

D'haeseleer E, Depypere H, Claeys S, Van Borsel J & Van Lierde KM (2009) 'The menopause and the female larynx, clinical aspects and therapeutic options: a literature review'. *Maturitas*, 64(1), pp. 27-32.

D'haeseleer E, Depypere H, Claeys S, Baudonck N & Van Lierde KM (2011) 'Vocal characteristics of middle-aged premenopausal women'. *Journal of Voice*, 23(3), pp. 360-6.

Ding H & Gray SD (2001) 'Senescent expression of genes coding collagens, collagen-degrading metalloproteinases and tissue inhibitor of metalloproteinases in rat vocal folds; comparison with skin and lungs'. *The Journals of Gerontology Series A: Biological Science and Medical Science*, 56(4), pp/ B145-52.

Dworkin JP, Reidy PM, Stachler RJ & Krouse JH (2009) 'Effects of sequential *Dermatophagoides pteronyssinus* antigen stimulation on anatomy and physiology of the larynx'. *Ear Nose and Throat Journal*, 88, pp. 793-99.

Ellis DA, Hopkin JM, Leitch AG & Crofton J (1979) 'Doctors' orders: controlled trial of supplementary, written information for patients'. *British Medical Journal*, 1, p. 456.

Enderby P & John A (2015) *Therapy Outcome Measures for Rehabilitation Professionals*, 3rd edn, J&R Press, Guildford.

Enderby P & John A (2019) *Therapy Outcome Measure User Guide*. J&R Press, Croydon.

Epstein R, Hirani SP, Stygall J & Newman SP (2009) 'How do individuals cope with voice disorders? Introducing the Voice Disability Coping Questionnaire'. *Journal of Voice*, 23(2), pp. 209-17.

Estill J (1988) *Belting and Classic Voice Quality: Some Physiological Differences. Medical Problems of Performing Artists*, Hanley and Belfus, Philadelphia, PA.

Fairbanks G (1960) *Voice and Articulation Drillbook*, 2nd edn, Harper & Bros, New York.

Fajt ML, Birnie KM, Bittar HE & Petrov AA (2018) 'Co-existence of VCD with pulmonary conditions other than asthma: a case series'. *Respiratory Medicine Case Reports*, 25, pp. 104-8.

Feretti R, Marques MJ, Khuran T & Neto HS (2015) 'Calcium buffering proteins in rat ILM'. *Physiology Reports*, 3(6), p. 12409.

Fex B, Fex S, Shiromoto O & Hirano M (1994) 'Acoustic analysis of functional dysphonia: before and after voice therapy (accent method)'. *Journal of Voice*, 8, pp. 163-7.

Firat Y, Engin-Ustun Y, Kizilay A, Akarcay M, Selinoglu E & Kafkasli A (2009) 'Level of intranasal estrogen on vocal quality'. *Journal of Voice*, 23(6), pp. 716-20.

Flodgren G, Rachas, A, Farmer AJ *et al.* (2015) 'Interactive telemedicine: effects on professional practice and health care outcomes'. *The Cochrane Database of Systemic Reviews*, 2015(9), CD002098.

Fontan L, Fraval M, Michon A, Déjean S & Welby-Gieusse M (2016) 'Vocal problems in sports and fitness instructors: a study of prevalence, risk factors, and need for prevention in France'. *Journal of Voice*, 31(2), p. 261.

Fowler SJ, Thurston A, Chesworth B *et al.* (2015) 'The VCDQ- a questionnaire for symptom monitoring in vocal cord dysfunction'. *Clinical and Experimental Allergy*, 45, pp. 1406-11.

Francis DO, Daniero JJ, Hovis KL *et al.* (2017) 'Voice related patient-reported outcome measure: a systematic review of instrument development and validation'. *Journal of Speech, Language and Hearing Research*, 60(1), 62-88.

Freidenberg CB (2002) 'Working with male-to-female transgendered clients: clinical considerations'. *Contemporary Issues in Communication Science and Disorders*, 29, pp. 43-58.

Fu S, Theodorus DG & Ward EC (2015) 'Delivery of intensive voice therapy for vocal fold nodules via telepractice: a pilot feasibility and efficacy study'. *Journal of Voice*, 29, pp. 696-706.

Gibbons N, Bray D & Harries M (2011) 'Long-term quantitative results of an Isshiki Type 4 thyroplasty'. *Journal of Voice*, 25(3), pp. 283-7.

Gibson PG & Vertigan AE (2015) 'Management of chronic refractory cough'. *British Medical Journal*, 351, p.h5590.

Gilman M, Merati AL, Klein AM, Hapner ER & Johns MM (2009) 'Performer's attitudes towards seeking health care for voice issues: understanding the barriers'. *Journal of Voice*, 23(2), pp. 225-8.

Greenhalgh T, Vijayaraghavan S, Wherton J *et al.* (2016) 'Virtual online consultations: advantages and limitations (VOCAL) study'. https://bmjopen.bmj.com/content/6/1/e009388.

Grillo EU (2017) 'An online telepractice model for the prevention of voice disorders in vocally healthy student teachers evaluated by a smartphone application'. *Perspectives of the ASHA Special Interest Groups*, 2(3), pp. 63-78.

Grillo EU, Brosious JN, Sorrell SL & Anand S (2016) 'Influence of smartphones and software on acoustic voice measures'. *International Journal of Telerehabilitation*, 8(2), pp. 9-14.

Guzman M, Laukkanen AM, Krupa P, Horacek J, Svec JG & Geneid A (2013) 'Vocal tract and glottal function during and after vocal exercising with resonance tube and straw'. *Journal of Voice*, 27(4), pp. 523.e19-523.e.34.

Haines J, Hull JH & Fowler SJ (2018), 'Clinical presentation, assessment and management of inducible laryngeal obstruction'. *Current Opinion in Otolaryngology & Head and Neck Surgery*, 26, pp. 174-9.

Halvorsen T, Walsted ES, Bucca C, Bush A, Cantarella G *et al.* (2017) 'ILO: an official joint European Respiration Society and European Laryngological Society Statement'. *European Respiratory Journal*, 50, 1602221.

Hamdan A-L, Mahfoud L, Sibai A & Seoud M (2009) 'Effect of pregnancy on the speaking voice'. *Journal of Voice*, 23(4), pp. 494-7.

Hammer MJ & Kruegar MA (2014) 'Voice related modulation of mechanosensory detection thresholds in the human larynx'. *Experimental Brain Research*, 232(1), pp. 13-20.

Hancock A, Oween K & Kissinger J (2010) 'Voice perceptions and quality of life of transgender people'. *Journal of Voice*, 25(5), pp. 553-8.

Hannu T, Saala E & Toskala E (2009) 'Long term prognosis of immediate hypersensitivity type of occupational laryngitis'. *Respiratory Medicine*, 103(1), pp. 130-5.

Harris T (1992) 'The pharmacological treatment of voice disorders'. *Folia Phoniatrica*, 44, pp. 143-54.

Hedge MN (2001) *Introduction to Communicative Disorders*, 3rd edn, Pro-Ed, Austin, TX.

Herrington-Hall B, Lee L, Stemple J, Niemi K & Miller-McHone M (1988) 'Description of laryngeal pathologies by age, sex and occupation in a treatment seeking sample'. *Journal of Speech & Hearing Disorders*, 53, pp. 57-64.

Heylen L (1997) *De Klinische Relevantie Van Het*, Fonetogram, Antwerp.

Hirano M (1981) *Clinical Examination of the Voice*, Springer-Verlag, New York.

Hirano M & Kurita S (1986) 'Histological structure of the vocal fold and its normal and pathological variation', in Kirschner JA (ed.), *Vocal Fold Histopathology*, College Hill Press, Baltimore, MA, pp. 17-24.

Hirano S, Minamiguchi S, Yamashita M, Ohno T, Kanemaru S & Kitamura M (2009) 'Histologic characterization of human scarred vocal folds'. *Journal of Voice*, 23(4), pp. 399-407.

Hogikyan ND & Sethuraman G (1999) 'Validation of an instrument to measure Voice-Related Quality of Life (V-RQOL)'. *Journal of Voice*, 13(4), pp. 557-69.

Howell S, Triptoli, E & Pring T (2009) 'Delivering the Lee Silverman Voice Treatment (LSVT) by web camera: a feasibility study'. *International Journal of Language and Communication Disorders*, 44(3), pp. 287-300.

Hunter EJ & Titze IR (2009) 'Quantifying vocal fatigue recovery: dynamic vocal recovery trajectories after a vocal loading exercise'. *Annals of Otolaryngology, Rhinology & Laryngology*, 118(6), pp. 449-60.

Isenberg JS, Crozier DL & Dailey SH (2008) 'Institutional and comprehensive review of laryngeal leukoplakia'. *Annals of Otolaryngology, Rhinology & Laryngology*, 117(1), pp. 74-9.

Jacobson BH, Johnson A, Grywalski C, Silbergleit A, Jacobson G, Benninger MS & Newman CW (1997) 'The Voice Handicap Index (VHI) development and validation'. *American Journal of Speech-Language Pathology*, 6(3), pp. 66-9.

John A, Enderby P & Hughes A (2005) 'Comparing outcomes of voice therapy: a benchmarking study using the therapy outcome measure'. *Journal of Voice*, 19(1), pp. 114-23.

Johnston BC, Ebrahim S, Carrasco-Labra Furukawa TA *et al.* (2015) 'Minimally important difference estimates and methods: a protocol'. *BMJ Open*, 5(1), e007953.

Jones SM (2016) *Laryngeal Endoscopy and Voice Therapy: A Clinical Guide*, Compton Publishing, Oxford.

Jones SM, Carding PN & Drinnan MJ (2006) 'Exploring the relationship between severity of dysphonia and voice-related quality of life'. *Clinical Otolaryngology*, 31(5), pp. 411-17.

Junuzovic Zunic L, Ibrahimagic A & Altumbabis S (2019) 'Voice characteristic in patients with thyroid disorders'. *The Eurasian Journal of Medicine*, 51(2), pp. 101-05.

Karatayli-Ozgursoy S, Pancheco-Lopez P, Hillel AT, Best SR, Bishop JA & Akst LM (2015) 'Laryngeal dysplasia, demographics and treatment a single institution review'. *JAMA Otolaryngology - Head & Neck Surgery*, 141(4), pp. 313-18.

Kempster GB, Gerratt BR, Verdolini Abbott K, Barkmeier-Kraemer J & Hillman RE (2009) 'Consensus auditory-perceptual evaluation of voice: development of a standardised clinical protocol'. *American Journal of Speech-Language Pathology*, 18, pp. 124-32.

Kessels RPC (2003) 'Patients' memory for medical information'. *Journal of the Royal Society of Medicine*, 96, pp. 219-22.

Khidr A, Noordzij JP, Meek R, Reibel JF & Levine PA (2003) 'Changes in the laryngeal signs of patients with reflux laryngitis; a prospective, placebo-controlled, randomized, double-blinded evaluation of omeprazole'. *Oto-Rhino-Laryngology Proceedings of the XVII World Congress of the IFOS*, 1240, pp. 843-51.

Kim HS, Moon JW, Chung SM & Lee JH (2011) 'Dysphonia in asthmatic patients'. *Journal of Voice*, 25(1), pp. 88-93.

Kiran S, Tandon U, Dwivedi D & Kumar R (2016) 'Prolonged hoarseness following endotracheal intubation - not so uncommon?' *Indian Journal of Anaesthesia*, 60(8), pp. 605-6.

Kloss JD & Lisman SA (2002) 'An exposure based examination of the effects of written emotional disclosure'. *British Journal of Health Psychology*, 7(pt1), pp. 31-46.

Kolbrunner J & Seifert E (2015) 'Encouragement to increase the use of psychosocial skills in the diagnosis and therapy of patients with functional dysphonia'. *Journal of Voice*, 31(I), pp. 132E1-132E7.

Kooijman PGC, De Jong FICRS, Oudes MJ, Huinck W, Van Acht H & Graamans K (2005) 'Muscular tension and body posture in relation to voice handicap and voice quality in teachers with persistent voice complaints'. *Folio Phoniatrica et Logopedics*, 57(3), pp. 134-47.

Kotby MN, El-Sady SR, Basiouny SE, Abou-Rass YA & Hegazi MA (1991) 'Efficacy of the accent method of voice therapy'. *Journal of Voice*, 5, pp. 316-20.

Koufman JA (1998) 'What are voice disorders and who gets them?' www.voiceinstituteofnewyork. com/who-gets-voice-disorders-and-why/.

Krätzig GP & Arbuthnott KD (2006) 'Perceptual learning style and learning proficiency: a test of the hypothesis'. *Journal of Educational Psychology*, 98, pp. 238-46.

Kreiman J & Gerratt BR (2011) 'Comparing two methods for reducing variability in voice quality measurements'. *Journal of Speech, Language and Hearing Research*, 54(3), pp. 803-12.

Kreiman J, Gerratt BR, Kempster GB, Erman A & Berke GS (1993) 'Perceptual evaluation of voice quality: review tutorial and a framework for future research'. *Journal of Speech and Hearing Research*, 36, pp. 21-40.

Kreiman J, Gerratt BR & Ito M (2007) 'When and why listeners disagree in voice quality assessment tasks'. *Journal of the Acoustical Society of America*, 122, pp. 2354-64.

Krisciunas GP, Vakharia A & Lazarus C (2019) 'Application of manual therapy for dysphagia in head and neck cancer patients: a preliminary national survey of treatment trends and adverse events'. Global Advances in Health and Medicine, 24(8), 2164956119844151.

Kummer AW (2020) 'Speech resonance disorders and velopharyngeal dysfunction (VPD)', in *Cleft Palate and Craniofacial Conditions: A Comprehensive Guide to Clinical Management*, 4th edn, Jones and Bartlett Learning, Burlington, MA.

LaGoria LA, Carnaby-Mann & Crary GD (2010) 'Treatment of vocal fold bowing using neuromuscular electrical stimulation'. *Archives of Otolaryngology – Head & Neck Surgery*, 136(4), pp. 398-403.

Law T, Lee K Y-S, Ho F, Vlantis A *et al.* (2012) 'The effectiveness of group voice therapy: a group climate perspective'. *Journal of Voice*, 26(2), pp. e41-e48.

Lee SW, Hong HJ, Seung HC & Doug IL (2014) 'Comparison of treatment modalities for contact granuloma – a national multi centre study'. *The Laryngoscope*, 124(5), pp. 1187-91.

Lenderking WR, Hillson E, Crawley JA, Moore D, Berzon R & Pashos CL (2003) 'The clinical characteristics and impact of laryngopharyngeal reflux disease on health-related quality of life'. *Value Health*, 6(5), pp. 560-5.

Liang FY, Huang XM, Chen L *et al.* (2017) 'Voice therapy effect on mutational falsetto patients: a vocal aerodynamic study'. *Journal of Voice*, 31, pp. 114.el-114.e5.

Lim JY, Lim SE, Choi SH, Kim JH, Kim KM & Choi HS (2007) 'Clinical characteristics and voice analysis of patients with mutational dysphonia: clinical significance of diplophonia and closed quotients'. *Journal of Voice*, 21, p. 12.

Lockhart M (2008) 'The breathing and voice workout'. Unpublished exercise programme.

Lockhart M (2009) 'Unpublished case studies of patients with aerophagia'.

Lockhart M (2011) 'Clinical efficiencies'. Presentation, AHP Advisory Committee, NHS Lanarkshire.

Long J, Williford HN, Olson MS & Wolfe V (1998) 'Voice problems and risk factors among aerobics instructors'. *Journal of Voice*, 12(2), pp. 197-207.

Ma EP & Yiu EM (2001) 'Voice activity and participation profile: assessing the impact of voice disorders on daily activities'. *Journal of Speech Language and Hearing Research*, 44(3), pp. 511-24.

Maclean N & Pound P (2000), 'A critical review of the concept of patient motivation in the literature on physical rehabilitation'. *Social Science & Medicine Group*, 50(4), pp. 495-506.

Maclean N, Pound P, Wolfe C & Rudd A (2000) 'Qualitative analysis of stroke patients' motivation'. *British Medical Journal*, 321, pp. 1051-4. 10.1136/bmj.321.7268.1051

Makdessian AS, Ellis DAF & Irish JC (2004) 'Informed consent in facial plastic surgery. Effectiveness of a simple educational intervention'. *Archives of Facial Plastic Surgery*, 6, pp. 26-30.

Malcomess K (2000) *'Delivering Clinical Governance in Speech and Language Therapy'*, TASLTM conference 'Countdown 2000', University of Edinburgh.

Malcomess K (2005) 'The Care Aims Model', in Anderson C & van der Gaag A (eds), *Speech and Language Therapy: Issues in Professional Practice*, Whurr, London.

Malcomess K (2015) 'The Care Aims Intended Outcomes Framework – Collaborative Decision-making for Well-being'. Blog, 12 June.

Malki KH, Nasser NH, Hassan SM & Farahat M (2008) 'Accent method of voice therapy for treatment of severe muscle tension dysphonia'. *Saudi Medical Journal*, 29(4), pp. 610-3.

Mallur PS & Rosen CA (2010) 'Vocal fold injection: review of indications, techniques, and materials for augmentation'. *Clinical and Experimental Otorhinolaryngology*, 3(4), pp. 177–82.

Marszalek S, Niebudek-Bogusz E, Woznicka E *et al.* (2012) 'Assessment of the influence of osteopathic myofascial techniques on normalization of the vocal tract functions in patients with occupational dysphonia'. *International Journal of Occupational Medicine and Environmental Health*, 25, pp. 225–35.

Martin S & Darnley L (1996) *The Teaching Voice*, Wiley Blackwell, Chichester.

Martin S & Darnley L (2019) *The Voice in Education*, Compton Publishing, Oxford.

Martin S & Lockhart M (2005) *The Voice Impact Profile*, Speechmark, Milton Keynes.

Maryn Y & De Bodt MS (2003) 'Ventricular dysphonia: clinical aspects and therapeutic options'. *The Laryngoscope*, 113(5), pp. 859–66.

Maryn Y, Corthals P, De Bodt M *et al.* (2009) 'Perturbation measures of voice; a comparative study between Multi-Dimensional Voice Programme and Praat'. *Folio Phoniatrica and Logopedics*, 61(4), pp. 217–26.

Mashima PA, Birkmire-Peters DP, Syms MJ, Holtel MR, Burgess LPA & Peters LJ (2003) 'Telehealth: voice therapy using telecommunications technology'. *American Journal of Speech-Language Pathology*, 12, pp. 432–39.

Maslan J, Leng X, Rees C, Blalock D & Butler SG (2011) 'Maximum phonation time in healthy older adults'. *Journal of Voice*, 25(6), pp. 709–13.

Matei A (2019) 'Shock horror! Do you know how much time you spend on your phone?' *The Guardian*, 21 August.

Mathieson L (1993) 'Vocal tract discomfort in hyperfunctional dysphonia'. *Journal of Voice*, 2, pp. 40–8.

Mathieson L (2001) *Greene and Mathieson's The Voice and its Disorders*, Wiley Blackwell, Chichester.

Mathieson L, Hirano SP & Epstein R (2007) The Vocal Tract Discomfort Scale. Available from voice-pathology@ucl.uk.

Mathieson L, Hirani SP, Epstein R, Baken RJ, Wood G & Rubin JS (2009) 'Laryngeal manual therapy: a preliminary study to examine its treatment effects in the management of muscle tension dysphonia'. *Journal of Voice*, 23(3), pp. 353–66.

Mattei A, Magalon J, Bertrand B, Philandrianos C, Veran J & Giovanni A (2017) 'Cell therapy and vocal fold scarring'. *European Annals of Otorhinolaryngology Head and Neck Diseases*, 134(5), pp. 339–45.

Meehan-Atrash J, Korzun T & Ziegler A (2019) 'Cannabis inhalation and voice disorders: a systematic review'. *JAMA Otolaryngology – Head & Neck Surgery*, 145(10), pp. 956–64.

Meerschman I, Van Lierde K, Ketels J *et al.* (2019) 'Effect of three semi-occluded vocal tract therapy programmes on the phonation of patients with dysphonia: lip trill, water resistance therapy and straw phonation'. *International Journal of Language and Communication Disorders*, 54(1), pp. 50–61.

Meurer EM, Garcez V, von Eye Corleta H & Capp E (2009) 'Menstrual cycle influences on voice and speech in adolescent females'. *Journal of Voice*, 23(1), pp. 109–13.

Miaskiewicz B, Szkielkowska A, Gos E, Panasiewicz A, Wtodarczyke E & Skarzynski PH (2018) 'Pathological sulcus vocalis – treatment approaches and voice outcomes in 36 patients'. *European Archives of Oto-Rhino-Laryngology*, 275(11), pp. 2763–71.

Miller T, Deary V & Patterson J (2014) 'Improving access to psychological therapies in voice disorders: a cognitive behavioural therapy model'. *Current Opinion in Otolaryngology – Head & Neck Surgery*, 22(3), pp. 2201–5.

Mordaunt M (2012) 'Summary', in Adler RK, Hirsh S & Mordaunt M (eds), *Voice and Communication Therapy for the Transgender/Transsexual Client*, Plural Publishing, San Diego, CA.

Morris MJ & Christopher KL (2010) 'Diagnostic criteria for the classification of vocal cord dysfunction'. *Chest*, 138(5), pp. 1213–23.

Morris RJ, Gorham-Rowan MM & Herring KD (2009) 'Voice onset time in women as a function of oral contraceptive use'. *Journal of Voice*, 23(1), pp. n4-18.

Morrison M & Rammage L (2000) *The Management of Voice Disorders*, Singular Publishing Group, San Diego, CA.

Morrison M, Rammage L & Emami AJ (1999) 'The irritable larynx syndrome'. *Journal of Voice*, 13(3), pp. 449-55.

Morton V & Watson DR (1998) 'The teaching voice:problems and perceptions'. *Logopedics Phoniatrics Vocology*, 23, pp. 133-9.

Moses PJ (1954) *The Voice of Neurosis*, Grune & Stratton, New York.

NCVS (2011) www.ncvs.org/research occu/html.

Neuenschwander MC, Sataloff RT, Abaza MM, Hawkshaw MJ, Reiter D & Spiegel JR (2001) 'Management of vocal fold scar with autologous fat implantation:perceptual results'. *Journal of Voice*, 15(2), pp. 295-304.

Nicolosi L, Harryman E & Kresheck J (2004) 'Terminology of communication disorders', in *Speech-Language-Hearing*, 5th edn, Lippincott Williams & Wilkins, Baltimore, MD.

Nixon I, Ramsay S & Mackenzie K (2010) 'Vocal function following discharge from intensive care'. *Journal of Laryngology and Otology*, 124(5), pp. 515-9.

Oates JM (2012) 'Evidence-based practice', in Adler RK, Hirsh S & Mordaunt M (eds), *Voice and Communication Therapy for the Transgender/Transsexual Client*, Plural Publishing, San Diego, CA.

Oates JM & Dacakis G (1983) 'Speech pathology considerations in the management of transsexualism - a review'. *British Journal of Disorders of Communication*, 18(3), pp. 139-51.

Ohno T, Hirano S & Rousseau B (2009) 'Age-associated changes in the expression and deposition of vocal fold collagen and hyaluronan'. *Annals of Otology, Rhinology & Laryngology*, 118(10), pp. 735-41.

Pannbacker M (1998) 'Voice treatment techniques; a review and recommendations for outcome studies'. *American Journal of Speech-Language Pathology*, 7(3), pp. 49-64.

Pasquale K, Wiatrack B, Woolley A & Lewis L (2009) 'Microdebrider versus CO2 laser removal of recurrent respiratory papillomas: a prospective analysis'. Presented at American Broncho-Esophagological Association COSDM, Orlando, FL, May 2000.

Patel RR, Bless DM & Thibeault SL (2011) 'Boot camp: a novel intensive approach to voice therapy'. *Journal of Voice*, 25(5), pp. 562-9.

Patel RR, Awan SN, Barkmeier-Kraemer *et al.* (2018) 'Recommended protocols for instrumental assessment of voice: American Speech-Language-Hearing Association Expert Panel to develop a protocol for instrumental assessment of vocal function'. *American Journal of Speech-Language Pathology*, 27, pp. 887-905.

Patrick DL, Burke LB, Powers MD *et al.* (2007) 'Patient-reported outcomes to support medical labeling claim: FDA perspective'. *Value in Health*, 10, Supplement 2.

Pau H & Murty GE (2001) 'First case of surgically corrected puberphonia'. *The Journal of Laryngology & Otology*, 115, pp. 60-1.

Pennebaker JW (1997) 'Writing about emotional experiences as a therapeutic process'. *Psychological Science*, 8, pp. 162-6.

Peterson-Falzone SJ, Trost-Cardamone JE, Karnell MP & Hardin-Jones MA (2017) *The Clinician's Guide to Treating Cleft Palate Speech*, 2nd edn, Elsevier, St Louis, MO.

Pham Q (2012) 'A randomised controlled trial comparing proton pump inhibitor therapy with and without interarytenoid Botulinum toxin injection for vocal fold granuloma'. Clinical Trials NCT, number NCT01678053.

Pham Q, Campbell R, Mattioni J & Sataloff R (2018) 'Botulinum toxin injections into the lateral cricoarytenoid muscles for vocal process granuloma'. *Journal of Voice*, 32(3), pp. 363-6.

Phillips PS *et al.* (2005), 'Does a specialist voice clinic change the ENT clinic diagnosis?' *Logopedics Phoniatrics Vocology*, 30, pp. 90-3.

Polanyi M (1967) *The Tacit Dimension*, Anchor Books, New York.

Preciado-Lopez J, Perez-Fernandez C, Calzada-Uriondo M & Preciado-Ruiz P (2008) 'Epidemiological study of voice disorders among teaching professionals of La Rioja, Spain'. *Journal of Voice*, 22(4), pp. 489–508.

Professional Studies Team (2010) 'Clinical thinking and management framework'. Unpublished education guide, Division of Language and Communication Science, City, University of London.

Puts DA, Hodges CR, Cárdenas RA & Gaulin SJC (2007) 'Men's voices as dominance signals: vocal fundamental and formant frequencies influence dominance attributions among men'. *Evolution and Human Behavior*, 28, pp. 340–4.

Radford R & Davies R (2020) 'Delivering voice therapy using Microsoft Teams@ RCSLT'. COVID-19 Telehealth webinar, 12 June.

Ramig LO & Verdolini K (1998) 'Treatment efficacy: voice disorders'. *Journal of Speech, Language and Hearing Research*, 41, pp. S101–16.

Ramig LO, Countryman S, O'Brien C, Hoehn M & Thompson I (1996) 'Intensive speech treatment for patients with Parkinson disease: short- and long-term comparison of two techniques'. *Neurology*, 47, pp. 1496–504.

Ramig LO, Sapir S, Countryman S, Pawlas A, O'Brien C, Hoen M & Thompson L (2001) 'Intensive voice treatment (LSVT®) for individuals with Parkinson's disease: a two year follow-up'. *Journal of Neurology, Neurosurgery & Psychiatry*, 71, pp. 493–8.

Randhawa PS, Mansuri S & Rubin JS (2009) 'Is dysphonia due to allergic laryngitis being misdiagnosed as laryngopharyngeal reflux?' *Logopedics, Phoniatrics, Vocology*, 35(1), pp. 1–5.

Rangarathnam B, McCullough G, Pickett H *et al.* (2015) 'Teleplactice versus in-person delivery of voice therapy for primary muscle tension dysphonia'. *American Journal of Speech Language Pathology*, 24(3), pp. 386–99.

Reeve BB, Wyrwich KW, Wu AW, Velikova G *et al.* (2013) 'ISOQOL recommends minimum standards for patient reported outcome measures used in patient centred outcomes and comparative effectiveness research'. *Quality of Life Research*, 22(8), pp. 1889–905.

Remacle M, Matar N, Morsomme D, Veduyckt I & Lawson G (2011) 'Glottoplasty for male to female transsexualism'. *Journal of Voice*, 25(1), pp. 120–3.

Rontal E, Rontal M, Jacob HJ & Rolnick MI (1979) 'Vocal cord dysfunction and industrial health hazard'. *Annals of Otolaryngology, Rhinology & Laryngology*, 88(1), pp. 818–21.

Roth D & Ferguson BJ (2010) 'Vocal allergy: recent advances in understanding the role of allergy in dysphonia'. *Current Opinion in Otolaryngology – Head and Neck Surgery*, 18(3), pp. 176–181.

Roy N & Ferguson NA (2001) 'Vowel formant changes following manual circumlaryngeal therapy for functional dysphonia: evidence of laryngeal lowering?' *Journal of Medical Speech-Language Pathology*, 9(3), pp. 169–75.

Roy N, Tasko SM & Harvey S (1995) 'Treatment results using the manual laryngeal musculoskeletal reduction procedure'. Paper presented at the convention of the American Speech-Language-Hearing Association, New Orleans, LA.

Roy N, Bless DM, Heisey D & Ford CN (1997) 'Manual circumlaryngeal therapy for functional dysphonia: an evaluation of short- and long-term treatment outcomes'. *Journal of Voice*, 11(3), pp. 321–31.

Roy N, Merrill RM, Thibeault S & Smith EM (2004) 'voice disorders in teachers and the general population: effects on work performance, attendance and future career choices'. *Journal of Speech, Language and Hearing Research*, 47, pp. 542–51.

Roy N, Nissen S, Dromey C & Sapir S (2009) 'Articulatory changes in muscle tension dysphonia: evidence of vowel space expansion following manual circumlaryngeal therapy'. *Journal of Communication Disorders*, 42(2), pp. 124–35.

Rubin AD, Hawkshaw MJ, Moyer CA, Dean CM & Sataloff RT (2005) 'Arytenoid cartilage dislocation: a 20 year experience'. *Journal of Voice*, 19, pp. 687–701.

Ryan M & Kenny D (2009) 'Perceived effects of the menstrual cycle on young female singers in the western classical tradition'. *Journal of Voice*, 23(1), pp. 99–108.

Sackley CM, Smith CH, Rick CE *et al.* (2018) 'Lee Silverman Voice Treatment versus control in Parkinson's disease: a randomized controlled trail (PDCOMM pilot)'. *Pilot and Feasibility Studies*, 4, p. 30.

Saeed AM, Riad NM, Osman NM, Nabil Khattab A *et al.* (2018) 'Study of voice disorders in patients with bronchial asthma and chronic obstructive pulmonary disease'. *The Egyptian Journal of Bronchology*, 12, pp. 20-6.

Salmen T, Ermakova T, Shindler A *et al.* (2018) 'Efficiency of microsurgery in Reinke's oedema evaluated by traditional voice assessment integrated with the Vocal Extent Measure (VEM)'. *Acta Otorhinolaryngologica Italica*, 38(3), pp. 194-203.

Sandlund C, Kane K, Ekstedt M *et al.* (2018) 'Patients' experiences of motivation, change and challenges in group treatment for insomnia in primary care: a focus group study'. *BMC Family Practitioner*, 19(1), p. 111.

Sato K & Hirano M (1997) 'Age-related changes of elastic fibres in the superficial layer of the lamina propria of vocal fold'. *Annals of Otolaryngology, Rhinology & Laryngology*, 106(1), pp. 44-8.

Sato K, Hirano M & Nakashima T (2002) 'Age related changes of collagenous fibres in the human vocal fold mucosa'. *Annals of Otology, Rhinology & Laryngology*, 111(1), pp. 15-20.

Sato K, Hirano M & Nakashima T (2017) '3D structure of the macula flava in the human vocal fold', in Sataloff RT (ed.), *Professional Voice*, 4th edn, Plural Publishing, Albany, NY.

Schindler A, Bottero A, Capaccio P, Ginocchio D, Adorni F & Ottaviani F (2008) 'Vocal improvement after voice therapy in unilateral vocal fold paralysis'. *Journal of Voice*, 22(1), pp. 113-8.

Schon DA (1983) *The Reflective Practitioner. How Professionals Think in Action*, Temple Smith, London.

Scott Howard N & Berke G (2012) 'Pediatric laryngeal disorders', in Shapiro N (ed.), *Handbook of Pediatric Otolaryngology*, World Scientific Publishing, Singapore, pp. 221-45.

Shah RK (2016) 'Acute laryngitis'. *Medscape*.

Shewell C (2009) *Voice Work: Art and Science in Changing Voices*, Wiley-Blackwell, Chichester.

Shulman GP, Holt NR, Hope DA, Mocarski R, Eyer J & Woodruff N (2017) 'Psychology of sexual orientation and gender diversity'. *Journal of the American Psychological Society*, 4(3), pp. 304-13.

Sidor M (2010) 'Laryngeal tremor clinical presentation'. Available from emedicine.medscape.com/article/867463-clinical.

Simberg S & Laine A (2007) 'The resonance tube method in voice therapy: description and practical implementations'. *Logopedics Phoniatrics Vocology*, 32, pp. 165-70.

Simberg S, Sala E, Tuomainen J, Sellman J & Rönnemaa AM (2006) 'The effectiveness of group therapy for students with mild voice disorders: a controlled clinical trial'. *Journal of Voice*, 20(1), pp. 97-109.

Simberg S, Sala E, Tuomainen J & Ronnemaa AM (2009) 'Vocal symptoms and allergy - a pilot study'. *Journal of Voice*, 23(1), pp. 136-9.

Slinger C, Mehdi SB, Milan SJ, Dodd S *et al.* (2019) 'Speech and language therapy for management of chronic cough'. *Cochrane Database of Systematic Reviews*, 2019(7), CD013067.

Smith S & Thyme K (1976) 'Statistic research on changes in speech due to pedagogic treatment (the Accent Method)'. *Folia Phoniatrica*, 28, pp. 98-103.

Snyder CF, Jensen R, Segal JB & Wu AW (2013) 'Patient-reported outcomes (PROs) putting the patient perspective in patient centred outcomes research'. *Medical Care*, 51(8), pp. S73-9.

Sodersten M, Hertegard S & Hammarberg B (1995) 'Glottal closure, transglottal airflow and voice quality in healthy middle aged women'. *Journal of Voice*, 9, pp. 182-97.

Song WJ, Chang YS, Faruqi S *et al.* (2015) 'The global epidemiology of chronic cough in adults: a systematic review and meta analysis'. *The European Respiratory Journal*, 45, pp. 1479-81.

Speyer R, Bogaardt HCA, Passos VL, Roodenburg NPHD *et al.* (2010) 'Maximum phonation time: variability and reliability'. *Journal of Voice*, 24(3), pp. 281-4.

Stanton K 'Mutational falsetto'. people.umass.edu.

Stemple J, Glaze L & Klaben BG (2013) *Clinical Voice Pathology: Theory and Management*, 5th edn, Plural Publishing, San Diego.

Stoneham G (2015) 'Sing for your life! Establishing a transgender voice group: benefits to students and clients'. *Proceedings of the European Professional Association of Transgender Health*, EPATH, Ghent.

Stoneham G and Mills M (2017) *The Voice Book for Trans and Non-Binary People: A Practical Guide to Creating and Sustaining Authentic Voice and Communication*, Jessica Kingsley, London.

Tateya I, Tateya T, Watanuki M & Bless D (2015) 'Homeostasis of hyaluronic acid in normal and scarred vocal Folds'. *Journal of Voice*, 29(2), pp. 133–9.

Tewfik TL (2011) 'Congenital malformations of the larynx', *Medscape Reference*.

Thyme-Frøkjær K & Frøkjær-Jensen B (2001) *The Accent Method, A Rational Voice Therapy in Theory & Practice*, Speechmark, Milton Keynes.

Titze IR (1994a) *Principles of Voice Production*, Prentice Hall, Englewood Cliffs, NJ.

Titze IR (1994b) 'Mechanical stress in phonation'. *Journal of Voice*, 8(2), pp. 99–105.

Titze IR (2001) 'Criteria for occupational risk in vocalisation', in Dejonckere PH (ed.), *Occupational Voice: Care and Cure*, Kugler Publications, The Hague.

Titze IR (2006) 'Voice training and theory with a semi-occluded vocal tract: rationale and scientific underpinnings'. *Journal of Speech, Language and Hearing Research*, 49(2), pp. 448–59.

Titze IR & Verdolini Abbott K (2012) *Vocology: The Science of and Practice of Voice Rehabilitation*, National Centre for Voice and Speech, Salt Lake City, UT.

Titze IR, Hunter EJ & Svec JG (2007) 'Voicing and silence in daily and weekly vocalizations of teachers'. *Journal of the Acoustical Society of America*, 121(1), pp. 469–78.

Towey MP (2012) 'Speech therapy telepractice for vocal cord dysfunction (VCD): MaineCare (Medicaid) cost savings'. *International Journal of Telerehabilitation*, 4(1), pp. 33–6.

Traister RS, Fajt ML & Petrov AA (2016) 'The morbidity and cost of VCD misdiagnosed as asthma'. *Allergy & Asthma Proceedings*, 37(2), pp. 25–31.

Tuomi L (2014) 'Voice outcome in patients treated for laryngeal cancer: efficacy of voice rehab'. *Journal of Voice*, 28, pp. 62–8.

Ullas G, McClellend L & Jones NS (2013) 'Medically unexplained symptoms and somatisation in ENT'. *Journal of Laryngology and Otolaryngology*, 127, pp. 452–7.

University of Iowa (2017) https://uiowa.edu/voice-academy.

Vaidya S & Vyas G (2006) 'Puberphonia: a novel approach to treatment'. *Indian Journal of Otolaryngology and Head and Neck Surgery*, 58, pp. 20–1.

Van Borsel J, de Pot K & De Cuypere G (2009) 'Voice and physical appearance in female-to-male transsexuals'. *Journal of Voice*, 23(4), pp. 494–8.

Van Gogh CDL, Verdonck-de Leeuw IM, Langerdijk JA *et al.* (2012) 'Long term efficacy of voice therapy in patients with voice problems after treatment of early glottic cancer'. *Journal of Voice*, 26, pp. 398–401.

Varma A, Agrahari AK, Kumar R & Kumar V (2015) 'Role of voice therapy in patients with mutational falsetto'. *International Journal of Phonosurgery and Laryngology*, 5(1), pp. 25–7.

Verdolini K (2000) 'Resonant voice therapy', in Stemple JC (ed.), *Voice Therapy: Clinical Case Studies*, 2nd edn, Singular, San Diego, CA.

Vertigan AE, Theodorus DG & Gibson PG (2006) 'Efficacy of speech pathology management for chronic cough: a randomised placebo controlled trial of treatment efficacy'. *Thorax*, 61(12), pp. 1065–9.

Ward PD, Thibeault SL & Gray SD (2002) 'Hyaluronic acid; its role in voice'. *Journal of Voice*, 16(3), pp. 303–9.

Watson PWB & McKinstry B (2009) 'A systematic review of interventions to improve recall of medical advice in healthcare consultations'. *Journal of the Royal Society of Medicine*, 102(6), pp. 235–43.

Whitling S, Lyberg-Ahlander V & Rydell R (2018) 'Absolute or relative rest after phonosurgery: a blind randomized prospective clinical trial'. *Logopedics, Phoniatrics, Vocology*, 43(4), pp. 143–54.

Willingham DT, Hughes EM & Dobolyi DG (2015) 'The scientific status of learning styles theories'. *Teaching of Psychology*, 42(3), pp. 266–71.

World Health Organization (1998) *A Health Telematics Policy in Support of WHO's Health-For-All Strategy for Global Health Development: Report of the WHO Group Consultation on Health Telematics*, WHO, Geneva.

World Health Organization (2001) *International Classification of Functioning, Disability and Health (ICF)*, WHO, Geneva.

World Health Organization (2008) *ICD-10 Classification of Mental and Behavioural Disorders*, WHO, Geneva.

Yamanaka H, Hayashi Y, Watanabe Y, Uematu H & Mashimo T (2009) 'Prolonged hoarseness and arytenoids cartilage dislocation after tracheal intubation'. *British Journal of Anaesthesia*, 103, pp. 452–5.

Yamasaki R, Behlau M, de Oliveira Campones do Brazil O & Yamashita H (2011) 'MRI anatomical and morphological differences in the vocal tract between dysphonic and normal adult women'. *Journal of Voice*, 25(6), pp. 743–50.

Yezdan F, Engin Ustun Kizilay A, Ustun Y, Akarcay M, Selimoglu E & Kafkasli A (2009) 'Effect of intranasal estrogen on vocal quality'. *Journal of Voice*, 23(6), pp. 716–20.

Yiu EM-L, Lo MCM & Barrett EA (2017) 'A systematic review of resonant voice therapy'. *International Journal of Speech and Language Pathology*, 19(1), pp. 17–29.

APPENDICES

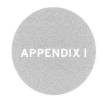

APPENDIX I

VOICE CARE RECOMMENDATIONS

In order to protect your voice, avoid:

- talking above loud background noise at social or sports events, or above office or machinery noise;
- smoking or vaping;
- chemical irritants and dusty conditions;
- recreational drugs;
- spicy foods and dairy products that may affect your voice;
- excessive use of the phone or mobile;
- drinks that cause dehydration, such as tea, coffee and carbonated soda drinks;
- dry atmospheres;
- eating a large meal just before going to bed at night as it may cause reflux;
- extensive voice use when emotionally challenged; the voice is closely linked with emotion and therefore vulnerable during times of tension, anxiety, depression or anger;
- whispering and continuing to talk if your voice is hoarse, or you are losing your voice.

Try to:

- keep alcoholic drinks to a minimum;
- be aware that hormonal changes such as the menopause, pregnancy or menstruation may affect voice quality;
- keep up your daily intake of water;
- be aware of the colour of your urine. Pale-coloured urine indicates an adequate level of hydration. However, some medication and food, such as beetroot, can alter the colour of urine;
- warm up the voice gently before prolonged speaking;
- use a humidifier or water spray to moisten the air in centrally heated offices or homes;

Copyright material from Stephanie Martin (2021), *Working with Voice Disorders*, Routledge

- keep physically fit and mobile in an effort to maintain effective respiration, reduce areas of tension and encourage vocal flexibility;
- get an adequate amount of sleep each night;
- take preventative measures to reduce the effect of allergies, irritants and changes to the mucosal lining of the nose and lungs, such as asthma;
- steam when required, particularly when ill and before prolonged periods of speaking;
- sip water or swallow if you feel you need to clear your throat as vigorous throat clearing can damage your vocal folds;
- monitor changes in your voice quality carefully and be aware of any increased tendency to cough or feeling dehydrated, particularly after changes to your medication;
- rest your voice when possible.

Copyright material from Stephanie Martin (2021), *Working with Voice Disorders*, Routledge

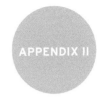

APPENDIX II

THE OCCUPATIONAL ENVIRONMENTAL AND ACOUSTIC CHECKLIST

OCCUPATIONAL ENVIRONMENTAL and ACOUSTIC CHECKLIST	YES	NO
Does your journey to and from work involve periods exposed to traffic fumes or poorly circulating air?		
Do you work in different physical spaces during the day? For example, do you move from indoors to outdoors?		
Is your workplace situated on or near a busy road/transport hub/building site?		
Is your workplace sited under an airport flight path?		
Do you work in a room with poor air quality for long periods of time?		
Is your workplace designated as open plan?		
Are you able to alter the room temperature at work?		
Are you in a dry atmosphere for a large part of the working day?		
Do you remain sitting or standing in one position for long periods of time while at work?		
Do you experience any physical discomfort such as back pain, stiff neck or shoulders as a result of your work?		
Is the acoustic environment given significance in your workplace?		
Do you work in a difficult acoustic environment?		
Does your workplace meet nationally recognised acoustic building regulations?		
Has there been an assessment of the acoustic properties of your workplace by a trained acoustician?		
Is there an auditory induction loop in your workplace?		
Have you been offered any advice regarding acoustic modification of your workplace to militate against vocal disorders?		
Do you feel you have sufficient voice rest periods during your working day?		
Would vocal strain be reduced by adaptations to your workplace		

Copyright material from Stephanie Martin (2021), *Working with Voice Disorders*, Routledge

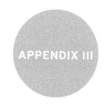

THE VOICE REVIEW CHECKLIST

Use this sheet to review how you have been feeling and what, if any, changes you have noticed that affected your voice during a specific time period

DATES FROM:	TO:		
During this period the quality of my voice has:		YES	NO
Remained the same			
Remained flexible			
Become increasingly strained			
Become more breathy			
Become increasingly husky			
Become more harsh			
Become lower in pitch			
Become higher in pitch			
Started to 'cut out' while I am speaking			

During this period I have:	YES	NO
Felt very tired		
Felt quite run down		
Felt not at all well		
Felt not very healthy		
Felt not at all energetic		
Had days off work through illness		
Remained very fit		
Remained energetic		
Remained very healthy		

Copyright material from Stephanie Martin (2021), *Working with Voice Disorders*, Routledge

During this period I have:	YES	NO
Felt quite stressed		
Felt generally quite anxious		
Felt depressed		
Felt generally quite angry		
Felt positive		
Felt quite calm		
Felt as though I could cope well at work and at home		
Not noticed any change in my emotional health		
Not noticed any sudden mood changes		

During this period I have:	YES	NO
Found it easy to make myself heard		
Found it difficult to make myself heard		
Found that sometimes my voice 'fades away' the longer I use it		
Found it difficult to change the volume of my voice		
Found it difficult to change the pitch of my voice		
Found that I have sometimes 'lost' my voice when speaking		
Found that I could not predict how my voice would sound when starting to speak		
Found that I often need to clear my throat when I am speaking		
Found that if I am speaking even for a short time I begin to cough		

Copyright material from Stephanie Martin (2021), *Working with Voice Disorders*, Routledge

During this period I have:	YES	NO
Tried to use my voice less		
Made changes to my diet		
Drunk more water		
Limited my alcohol intake		
Cut down on cigarettes		
Warmed up vocally		
Made time to complete my daily voice diary		
Limited my time in noisy, dry or dusty environments		
Steamed		

Any additional comments:

Copyright material from Stephanie Martin (2021), *Working with Voice Disorders*, Routledge

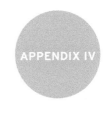

APPENDIX IV

VOICE DIARY

	Morning	Afternoon	Evening	Overall Voice Quality
Monday				
Tuesday				
Wednesday				
Thursday				
Friday				
Saturday				
Sunday				

Please complete every section of this chart each day using the following scale:

1 = Voice rest 2 = Easy voicing 3 = Possible vocal stress 4 = Vocal loading

Copyright material from Stephanie Martin (2021), *Working with Voice Disorders*, Routledge

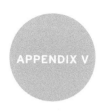

CASE HISTORY PROFORMA

Name _____   No. of adults in home _____

Address _____   No. of children in home _____

_____   Relationships of those in home _____

Date of birth _____   Closest relative/Significant other

Family doctor _____   _____

ENT consultant _____

Hospital/Unit No. _____

REFERRAL DETAILS

Referral agent	Referral diagnosis

ENT REPORT

Indirect laryngoscopy	Ears/Hearing
Videostroboscopy	Nose/Sinuses/Pharynx
Oral Cavity/Hygiene/Dentition	Naso-pharyngeal sphincter

THE VOICE DISORDER

Onset of dysphonia	Severity, duration and frequency of dysphonia episodes
The pattern of voice disturbance	Previous episodes of therapy
Patient's perception of voice disorder	Clinician's perception of voice disorder

Copyright material from Stephanie Martin (2021), *Working with Voice Disorders*, Routledge

MEDICAL HISTORY

Previous illnesses/Surgery	Medication
Upper respiratory tract	Allergies/Viral infections
Asthma/Use of inhalers	Back pain/Joints/Posture
Digestion/Diet Drugs/	Smoking/Alcohol/Recreational Caffeine
Chronic fatigue/Recurring viral illness	Stress-related illness/Emotional fragility

EMPLOYMENT

Acoustics/Noise levels	Use of protective equipment/Amplifiers
Ventilation/Heating/Pollution	Hours/Conditions
Postural demands	Training for vocal loading

DOMESTIC/SOCIAL/RECREATIONAL ACTIVITIES

Domestic	Social and recreational activities

GENERAL COMMENTS

Copyright material from Stephanie Martin (2021), *Working with Voice Disorders*, Routledge

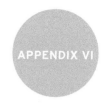

APPENDIX VI

VOICE ASSESSMENT SHEET

Name	Hospital/Unit No.
Address	
Date of birth	
Date of assessment	**Assessed by**
Posture	Seated Standing
Breathing method	
Degree of general body tension	
Degree of specific body tension	
Tongue, jaw and neck tension	
Laryngeal and pharyngeal tension	
Vocal attack	
Vocal support	
Phonation time	
Production of reflexive sounds	
Pitch/voice placement	
Voice projection	
Severity rating	
Vocal quality	
Articulatory precision	
Resonance	
Additional comments	

Copyright material from Stephanie Martin (2021), *Working with Voice Disorders*, Routledge

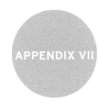

APPENDIX VII

PROGNOSTIC INDICATOR CHECKLIST

Prognostic Indicator	Positive	Negative
Normal larynx		
Prognosis for laryngeal recovery		
Possible aetiological factors		
Contributing factors:		
General health		
Hearing acuity		
Environmental/occupational factors		
Personal factors		
Duration of the voice disorder		
Degree to which the voice disorder affects the patient:		
Impairment		
Disability		
Handicap		
Well-being		
Would the patient improve with advice only?		
Is the patient well motivated for change?		
Is this a realistic expectation?		
Will the patient receive positive support:		
From family/significant others?		
At work?		
Have there been previous episodes of the voice disorder?		
Is this the same disorder?		
Has the patient had voice therapy before?		
Was it successful?		
Was it unsuccessful?		

Copyright material from Stephanie Martin (2021), *Working with Voice Disorders*, Routledge

Index

Note: Page numbers in **bold** indicate tables, and in *italics* indicate figures.